Following the Great Physician

The First 70 Years
of the
Christian
Medical & Dental
Associations

ISBN 0-9706631-0-2

Library of Congress Control Number: 2002106511

Manufactured in the United States of America
by Central Plains Book Manufacturing, Winfield, Kansas

Table of Contents

Introduction
Acknowledgements
Foreword by Dr. David Stevens
Message from Dr. Alva B. Weir, III
Dedication

Appendix

Introduction

*I*n the early 90s, General Director Hal Habecker asked us to help research and tell the story of the organization now known as the Christian Medical & Dental Associations (CMDA). As we reviewed materials and talked to members, it wasn't long before we saw that the main thread through all the years was God's hand in and through the organization. Interviews with long-time members, many of them former leaders, consistently testified not to their own wisdom or skills, but to the grace and faithfulness of God.

Through the years, CMDA has had several names, the first being CMS—the Christian Medical Society. In 1988, the name was changed to CMDS—the Christian Medical & Dental Society, more accurately identifying what had been for years a ministry to and with physicians and dentists. The change to CMDA occurred in 2000. So one challenge for us, in writing about seventy years of ministry, was how to refer to the organization, which had remained true to its calling whatever name it employed. Our solution was to use the name used in the era being described in a given chapter.

Speaking of names, another challenge was knowing how to properly refer to those with various degrees, including those with various non-doctoral graduate degrees and those with doctorates in a non-medical or dental field. Where possible, we have identified the degrees of these—usually staff members—and others at least once in the text, usually when they are first mentioned. However, it was not possible for us to discover the professional degrees of all mentioned in the book, so when their degree was not known, we have included them by name as a way of honoring their contribution as opposed to leaving them out because we could not discover the correct initials to use after their names. We trust that none of these servants of CMDA will be offended by this decision.

In the case of those with doctorates in the fields of medicine, dentistry, or psychology, we have usually referred to them as "doctor," in some cases including their specific degrees or a reference in the text identifying their field.

Perhaps our greatest challenge was knowing that many stories that could have been included remained unknown to us, in part because so many have served quietly, with no desire for recognition. We regret that we could not mention many people who have been involved, because of limited space. But it is good to know that the God who raised up this organization for such a time as this has taken note of them all.

Dr. John Elsen, President of CMS in 1948, wrote a letter in 1999, excerpted in *Today's Christian Doctor.* He said, "Remembering the past is only of value if it points us to likewise take up the torch and run the race that the Lord has given us. And the Lord remembers even the things we forget about His servants."

As a result of our research, we are all the more aware of the "great cloud of witnesses" who, like those in Hebrews 11, have gone before us. We have read of them, sometimes through worn-out, hard-to-decipher copies of minutes of early meetings. What a respect we have gained for them as they "ran the race set before them," through good times and hard times, struggles and victories, with vision and determination to carry out God's work in and through the medical and dental professions.

We, like you, look forward to great days ahead for the Christian Medical & Dental Associations. May this history remind us to remain faithful to the God whose work this is.

Dr. Bob and Marian Schindler
Ephesians 3: 20, 21

Acknowledgements

Many people helped us tell this seventy-year-long story. We thank them for the tremendous part they have played in making it live today for the readers.

It was General Director Hal Habecker who called us in the early '90s and asked if we would help in writing the history of (at that time) CMDS. Thank you, Hal, for your burden for the need to preserve history, and for your encouragement to us. We are only sorry that it has taken this long to finish the project.

A special thanks to Dr. Richard Gieser, who has a heart for the history, as his father was a founder. He loaned us material for the book and cheered us on.

A word of appreciation for the present leadership—Executive Director Dr. David Stevens and the CMDA Trustees—who have greatly encouraged us and said it was time to finish it now. We needed a deadline!

Our thanks to Tracie Coppedge, Executive Assistant to our CMDA Executive Director, Dr. David Stevens, who amid her very busy work schedule, responded to our request for someone in the Bristol office to write the closing chapters from the '90s on through 2001. We knew that so many great things have happened in those years, and who better could tell it? She did a tremendous job.

David Biebel, D. Min., Editor of Today's Christian Doctor and former field staff member, is himself an author, and he was a great help in editing this history. It was an asset that he is familiar with the ministry of CMDA and has a passion to tell the story, too. Thank you, Dave. We'll miss your frequent e-mails!

Our appreciation also goes to Glenn F. Arnold, Ph.D., who helped with early editing on the first chapters. He has been head of the Communications Department at Wheaton College Graduate School, as well as at Moody Bible Institute. Dr. Richard Gieser put us in touch as we began writing.

Barbara Snapp, Paul Tournier Institute's Academic Liaison at CMDA, coordinated it all as the manuscripts and pictures were sent to her. She knew how to keep track of all the details for publishing. And we never heard a sign of frustration! She was great. And she was ably assisted with the design of the book by CMDA graphic designers Alison Turner and Jay Huron. And a special thanks goes to Mike Wilson of B&B Printing in Bristol, Tennessee, for help with the cover design.

Our appreciation goes to all who were willing to tell your story to us, through interviews and through publications. You were there when it happened, and so you helped to put it all together.

"To God be the glory, great things He has done,"
Dr. Bob and Marian Schindler

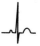

Foreword

by David Stevens, M.D.

One of the mysteries of God's grace is that He deigns to work through men and women to build His kingdom. I'm amazed that He doesn't look for people with certain abilities or accomplishments. Instead, He looks for those who have willing hearts and teachable spirits that seek Him above all.

On our seventieth birthday, we do well to look back and remember our roots. It is a time to recall those men and women who sacrificially built an organization that today enjoys national and international impact.

Yet, if we asked them, they would say that the Christian Medical & Dental Associations was not their ultimate goal. Their real goal was to invest their lives in the lives of others. They wanted to bring people to Christ and honor God in all that they did. They wanted to understand, from the Great Physician's point of view, what it really means to be a Christian doctor. They wanted to personally strive to become that ideal and challenge other doctors and students to do the same. CMDA was then, and is today, only a means to an end.

As we look back, we can more clearly see God's purpose, plan, and faithfulness. Little did our founding fathers realize the great expansion of medical missions that would take place after WWII or the critical role CMDA would play in challenging, educating, and equipping healthcare missionaries around the world. They couldn't foresee remarkable scientific advances, enhanced technologies, or that there would need to be a professional Christian voice to speak out on ethical issues from abortion to genetic determinism.

God had a plan, when He started with one medical student in Chicago praying in his top bunk bed, to build a nationally successful ministry of approximately 16,000 members to meet the challenges of today. Throughout the history of our organization there have been crises and trials, yet in the midst of every difficulty, God has demonstrated His faithfulness.

I'm so glad that even though there is an end to this fascinating chronicle of CMDA's history, God's purpose, plan, and faithfulness still continue. We can't predict what is ahead in medicine and dentistry, but we do know that we are in the midst of a storm. Raging seas are eroding the foundations of our professions. The winds of managed care, the lightning of malpractice, and the whirlpools of ethical issues buffet us from every side.

Looking back at our history, with the help of this book, reminds me that God does His best work in crises. His purposes will not be thwarted. God doesn't have problems; He only has plans. He has been faithful, and He will not fail us in the days ahead. Being reminded of these truths transforms my fears and anxiety into praise and thanksgiving. That alone makes the following pages well worth the read.

David Stevens, M.D.

A Message from CMDA President
Alva B. Weir III, M.D.

Greatness comes in a variety of packages: there's the George Washington package, the Billy Graham package, the missionary doctor package and the Mother Teresa package. But there are many more.

Recently, I attended the birthday party of a 79-year-old Christian doctor. It was a simple affair with good food, bad jokes, and an air filled with memories. This doctor is a great man who continues to practice medicine with patients who have been helped by his heart and skills for decades. He is still as sharp as a suture needle and has more energy than I ever had, even in my youth. He is a great man.

Some Christian doctors find their greatness in organizations, or in great academic discovery, or in years of sacrificial service to the poor. Their greatness lies where God has placed them and comes because they are willing to follow Him there. This particular doctor has spent over fifty years in a private/academic practice in Memphis, Tennessee, and is great for the same reason. Over the years I have watched him and learned.

He has pursued excellence in medicine: God called him to do his best for the people placed before him.

He has been selfless in his care: money was never the goal; sleep was never the priority.

He has the touch of kindness; he has the coldest hands and warmest heart of any man I know.

He has shared his wisdom eagerly: always the teacher; always the encourager.

He has never sought the praise of man, though he has received it a hundred thousand times from the lips of his patients.

He has remained faithful to his family and church in a world that cares little for either.

He has walked hand in hand with Jesus, never approaching a patient or a colleague without the Master at his side.

He has persevered; he has continued to accomplish the work to which God has called him day after day, year after year. What can he do of greater value? He is a Christian doctor.

I write of this man not so much as a memorial to my father but as a standard to raise high and to follow—the standard of a Christian doctor. This man is great because he has walked the walk of Christ. He is great because he has been faithful to his calling. His actions have manifested the touch of Jesus one act at a time, one patient at a time, throughout a lifetime. He is a Christian doctor.

My head is filled with dreams of great things that I might do for God and man. I would gladly trade them all if I could become the doctor that my father has been.

Alva B. Weir III, M.D.

P.S. In the pages of this book, you'll read many names of those who have accomplished great things within the context of CMDA. Due to space limitations, you'll not read of the many others, who, like my father, have accomplished a simpler greatness, yet one with eternal recognition: "Well done, good and faithful servant." Thankfully, the only One who says this keeps the only Book that matters.

Dedication

*T*his book is dedicated to its primary authors, Dr. Bob and Marian Schindler, who tirelessly pursued every detail and available photo for months, soliciting salient quotes and tracking down pertinent facts like detectives on assignment. The result shows that they were the perfect choice to produce this volume.

The Schindlers became officially involved with CMDA with Bob's student membership in 1954. During their thirteen years in Liberia (1962-75), Bob founded and directed the medical program at ELWA Hospital. Both Bob and Marian were honored by the Liberian government—Bob as a "Knight Great Band, Humane Order of African Redemption," and Marian as a "Knight Official." Together they authored the book, *Mission Possible*, using their experiences as a backdrop.

From 1983-1988, Bob was a member of the Board of Trustees, serving CMDA as President from 1985-1987. As a result of a conversation with CMS Mexico's president just after Bob had handed the gavel to Dr. Mayo Gilson in 1987, both Bob and Marian led the way in launching a whole new arm of CMDA's outreach, the Commission on International Medical Educational Affairs (COIMEA), which they led until their "retirement" as co-administrators on December 31, 2000. COIMEA's goal was to reach national physicians and dentists in their own countries by sending Christian educator-doctors who would go at their own expense to demonstrate the latest techniques, while forming relationships that might lead to discussions of matters of faith. Perhaps as a result of their world-wide friendship circle, Bob was elected as President of the International Christian Medical & Dental Association in 1998.

The key word in the Schindlers' life has been relationship. In everything they've done, they've sought to bring others—patients and colleagues—to a personal relationship with Jesus Christ, their own Savior and role model. As the citation of their 1996 "Servant of Christ Award" from CMDA acknowledged, of all their awards and recognitions, their ultimate honor has been to touch as many people as possible for the Lord.

The following CMDA members expressed, in behalf of themselves and the organization, a sense of appreciation for Bob and Marian, which words can hardly articulate:

"I first met Bob Schindler when he was a fourth-year medical student…. My admiration for him and Marian is boundless. Their devotion, service, and love for others marks their ministry to this day."
—Richard Topazian, D.D.S.

"Bob and Marian both mentor with humor, humility, and with Christ's love."
—Jon Askew, M.D.

"We love you, and wish you God's blessings. May all you have mentored carry on your work and pass it on to another generation."
—Warren Heffron, M.D.

"Bob and Marian Schindler are the best example of a husband and wife ministry team that I know. They have been a shining example to me as I make my way along the pilgrimage known as the Christian life."
—Jeffrey J. Barrows, D.O.

"Bob and Marian Schindler were my father and mother in medical missions. They are visionaries who could always see beyond the horizon. They served and 'saw' with the eyes of faith, a very big God who could be relied upon to perform miracles with regularity. They had infectious enthusiasm for serving others of all stations in life through their medical expertise and through their friendship evangelism. They loved people where the people were at and also for what they believed they could become in Christ."
—David E. Van Reken, M.D.

"As a younger professional, I have known Bob and Marian since my childhood. They project the belief that each idea can be investigated. They never discouraged pursuing my ideas of opportunities. They lead by example and continue to encourage what can be done—for in Christ, all things are possible."
—Neal Smith, D.D.S.

"Bob and Marian have been, and are, good friends. Bob is a great mentor and exhorter. I learned a lot from my association with him on the Board of Trustees."

—Mayo D. Gilson, M.D.

"Bob and Marian have touched and influenced so many lives. They jump-started my involvement with COIMEA by giving me $500 to go to the Philippines. Their book on missions is a classic still, and has deeply influenced me, personally."

—Donald Wood, M.D.

"No couple better personifies a life of sacrificial service to the Lord. Their ministry has spanned the globe and touched lives next door. CMDA would not be where it is today without the many contributions of the Schindlers."

—David Stevens, M.D.

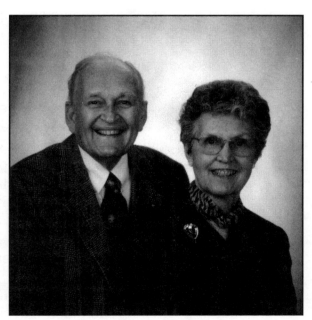

Bob and Marian Schindler

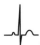

Chapter 1
The Birth of the Society:
The 1930s

*L*oneliness hung heavy in George Peterson's room in a fraternity house in 1931. George was a first-year student at Northwestern University Medical School in Chicago. In his first days at Northwestern, he was very sensitive about being a country boy from Wisconsin, living in a big city for the first time. He felt that he had no real friends with whom to share his sense of isolation. On his desk among the medical books stood his Bible and a copy of the devotional book, *Streams in the Desert*.

One evening, early in that freshman year, a second-year student came to George's room and introduced himself. He was Kenneth Gieser, who had decided to visit the first-year students on the third floor of his Phi Beta Pi House. As conversation began about their studies, Ken suddenly spotted the devotional book.

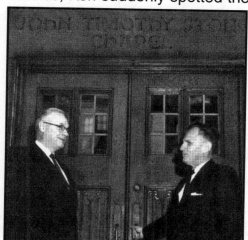

Dr. George A. Peterson and Dr. P. Kenneth Geiser visiting the John Timothy Stone Chapel, where CMS was founded.

Picture: © American Medical Association, Today's Health, Mar. 1965/Courtesy AMA Archives

"George, how come you have *Streams in the Desert* on your desk? This is the first time I've seen that book in this house!"

"Well, sir, I just happen to be a Christian and I read this along with my Bible every day," George replied in his matter-of-fact way.

"You're my kind of a man, George. I've been waiting for you." With that, Ken quickly switched the conversation to their common faith. They joyfully discovered that they were brothers in Christ.

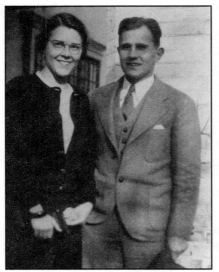

Kay and Kenneth Gieser at the home of Dr. & Mrs. L. Nelson Bell in Tsing Kiang Pu, October 1934.

The previous year—with very few Christian friends—Kenneth Gieser had also found his first months of medical school extremely lonesome. At night, he often crawled into his upper bunk to pray: "Lord, I'm so bewildered I can't seem to think straight anymore. Hold me until I can get out of this materialistic situation and can breathe in clear fresh air once again."

Gieser had found that this was an era when a Christian in science or medicine was an oddity, and there was a struggle to keep the faith. But after his visit with Peterson, he was encouraged.

The men determined to meet regularly for Bible reading and prayer. The small John Timothy Stone Chapel in Chicago's Fourth Presbyterian Church on Michigan Avenue became their special sanctuary every Saturday noon. Dr. Gieser recalled, years later: "George and I found that we could meet there on Saturdays after classes. We would read a portion of Scripture together, and then each of us prayed. Though we only spent a very few minutes together, this was a great time of spiritual strengthening and renewal. Soon others joined us." The John Timothy Stone Chapel became the birthing room for the Christian Medical Society, or CMS, as it was called for many years.

By 1932, the meeting place had moved a few blocks south to the Lawson YMCA so that they could meet for lunch. Three years later, the number of participants had increased to fifteen, when a group started at the University of Illinois Medical School by Franklin A. Olson joined with those at Northwestern University.

Everett Nicholas joined the group when he entered Northwestern in '35. He found the fellowship so important that he said, "I rarely missed a meeting in four years. In all, that would be about 150 meetings!" He recalls that many others also were regular in attendance. "Even Henry Schweinfurth, who worked as a night elevator operator, came when he could," Dr. Nicholas said.

It was a close-knit group, but there was no formal organization until the 1934-35 school year, when a constitution was written and the first officers were elected. The group named itself the Christian Medical Society. The constitution stated these objectives of the Society:

> To provide and foster Christian fellowship among the members of the medical schools and the profession through weekly meetings for reading and discussion of the Bible and for prayer, to be supplemented by outside speakers, and to present a positive witness of God our Father and our Savior Jesus Christ to the medical profession.

Membership was based on profession of the Christian faith as stated in Romans 10:9 and majority vote of the members present at a specified meeting. Seventeen signatures were attached, along with those of six honorary members. The first president and vice-president—Franklin A. Olson and Henry Schweinfurth—were both medical students.

Informal get-togethers occurred in the corner of the graduate assistants' chemistry laboratory at Northwestern. Jonathan Cilley and Joe Boutwell, both working on their Ph.D.'s in physiological chemistry, were to play a significant role in the development of CMS. Dr. John Frame recalls:

> While in medical school, I would eat with them at the corner of the lab. My standard lunch was two peanut butter and grape jelly sandwiches, a glass of milk and an orange—the cheapest well-balanced meal I could get. In addition there was a famous supper to which wives, sweethearts, and fiancées were invited, and we all contributed.

There was a bit of excitement when one of the women asked Joe where the milk was kept. He told her: "the second refrigerator." There was a scream when she opened the door to find a dead dog. Joe had neglected to tell her whether it was in the upper or lower fridge!

The spouses helped with the organization, too. Dr. Everett Nicholas remembers that his sister, Dorothy, who later became the wife of Dr. Jonathan Cilley, and Dr. John Hyde's wife, Virginia, kept the Society's records in a shoebox for awhile.

Foreign missions were a big part of the vision of those young men in the early days. According to an article written by Dr. Gieser for the Northwestern University Medical School magazine, out of the small group that met for fellowship in the early '30s, a significant number went to the mission field from Northwestern: Douglas Parker ('32) to China, Robert Hockman ('32) to Ethiopia, Frank Pickering ('33) to Peru, Edward Pain ('33) to Ethiopia, Kenneth Gieser ('34) to China, and Robert Sandilands ('35) to Africa.

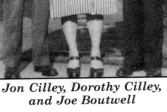

Jon Cilley, Dorothy Cilley, and Joe Boutwell

Dr. Kenneth Gieser is credited with being the founder of the Society. But after 1934, he was not able to stay in Chicago to help in those early years. As a premedical student at Wheaton College, he had heard Dr. E. R. Kellersberger of the American Mission to Lepers challenge the students to give their lives for missionary service. This challenge spoke directly to Ken. He had come to medical school with a vision for the mission field, and specifically to take his practice to Africa.

In his senior year in medical school, Ken married Kay Kirk, a former classmate at Wheaton. As they looked forward to Ken's internship at West Suburban Hospital in Oak Park, Illinois, they also sent inquiries to different mission boards working in Africa, but they received no encouragement. This was in 1934, when the nation was beginning to recover from the Great

4

Depression, and not many missions were sending out missionaries at that time. One board did say, however, that they had just received a cablegram from Dr. L. Nelson Bell in China. Dr. Bell had been given a special grant, and he wanted an intern for the coming year to serve with him at the 400-bed Tsing Kiang Pu Presbyterian Hospital in Kiangsu Province.

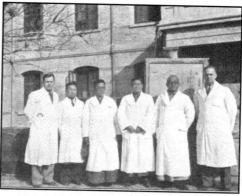

T.K.P. staff doctors Geiser, Kok, Tsoa, Wu, Chien and Bell in 1938.

Ken said to Kay, "If there is any place we don't want to serve, it's China. But probably the Lord will send us there."

Within a short time, all the obstacles—among them that Dr. Gieser would need to be released from his internship contract; that if he were to intern outside the United States, the hospital would have to be recognized by both Northwestern and the AMA; and, that he would have to take the state Boards before leaving—had been worked out.

So in August 1934, Dr. and Mrs. Kenneth Gieser sailed to China, where Dr. Gieser worked alongside missionary-statesman Dr. L. Nelson Bell (father of Ruth Bell Graham) for the next six years. Dr. Bell was a skilled surgeon, and Dr. Gieser loved the mornings filled with surgery. Ken and Kay also enjoyed the Bells' warmth and their joy in serving Christ. The Bells became their spiritual mentors.

However, just a few years after arriving in China, the Giesers saw their world there beginning to collapse. These were very troublesome times as the Japanese took over the city of Tsing Kiang Pu in 1939. Dr. Gieser also became seriously ill with two types of malaria and pneumonia, and they had to return to the States in 1940. The doctors advised him not to return to the mission field because of his health. An ophthalmology residency opened for him at the University of Illinois in Chicago.

During Dr. Gieser's absence, unknown to him and other initiators of the Chicago area CMS effort, similar developments were happening in Philadelphia, where in 1935 several medical students had asked noted minister Dr. Donald Grey Barnhouse to conduct a Bible study for them. For the next four years, these students met with Dr. Barnhouse every Monday morning at seven o'clock, until by 1939 the group averaged approximately ten in number.

Also in Philadelphia, perhaps beginning as early as 1937, some of the graduate physicians began meeting for Bible study and prayer one Sunday afternoon a month. Although these meetings were temporarily discontinued with the advent of the Second World War, they were reinstated with fervor after the war ended.

In 1939 a significant effort was made to expand CMS. From just ten square feet of desktop and locker space in the Northwestern lab, the group rented a post office box, got a permit, and sent cards to all incoming freshmen students at Northwestern University and the University of Illinois Medical Schools, inviting them to the CMS meetings. Dr. Frame recalls that, "Out of a hundred twenty incoming freshmen, we had something like ten or twelve responses showing interest in our group, and about half of these became active."

The initial response was small, but the vision to reach out had been launched, and CMS was beginning to grow. The Society began to hear reports of other Christian groups meeting in medical schools in other parts of the country. The Society members hoped that one day all these groups could interact and fellowship with one another.

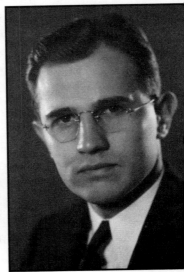

For each decade there have been challenges and opportunities for the unique Christian organization that began with Kenneth Gieser's visit to George Peterson's room in his fraternity house in 1931.

Kenneth Gieser

Dr. Gieser's influence on the Christian Medical Society continued through the years until his death in 1987. In a letter to membership at the 50th Anniversary of CMS, Dr. Gieser recounted his greatest desires for CMS:

> **First,** that we remain true to the faith once delivered and to the purposes for which we were organized.

> **Second,** that we become more emboldened in our outreach...we need to become more proficient in our personal witness for Christ in order to serve both the physical as well as the spiritual needs of people.

> **Third,** that we enthusiastically support CMS with our fervent prayers and generous financial support.

Chapter 2
Expansion and Organization:
The 1940s

*B*y the early 1940s, Christian medical groups had formed in Chicago, Philadelphia, and New York—at Columbia University College of Physicians and Surgeons (P&S). It was from the latter group that the Chicago CMS received its first call for help. "We are inclined to feel that our most urgent responsibility is to present to the non-Christian students of our own school the Gospel," the representative wrote. "This year has seen the beginning of an organized program for this purpose at P&S, with a meeting every two weeks led by an evangelical Christian speaker who is able to talk the language which the students understand."

In 1941 George Kollmar, a P&S student, wrote to say that he was meeting with three other Christian students, but they wanted advice on a doctrinal statement for membership for their group. They wanted to remain evangelical in the midst of a growing atmosphere of liberalism among organizations. Could CMS help? Would it even be possible to join with the Chicago society?

These calls for help forced the Chicago group to move more quickly to form a constitution and a statement of belief for a national CMS. A committee of four had already been working on this—Joe Boutwell and Jonathan Cilley (both graduate students at Northwestern), John Frame (a missionary kid and a medical student at Northwestern) and Brad Steiner (also a son of missionaries and a medical student at the University of Illinois). In January 1942 the committee in Chicago wrote to George Kollmar:

> As you will see from the enclosed report, we had had a plan for a national organization for two years but it had not seemed proper to introduce it.... We received your letter just as the committee was meeting to consider this so we knew that we had additional reasons; therefore, we are sending copies of the 'Constitution' to you and several other groups for consideration.

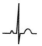

The statement of faith, which individual applicants for membership in the national Christian Medical Society were asked to sign, read:

I believe:

> *In the verbal inspiration, original inerrancy, and final authority of the Bible.*
>
> *In the unique deity of our Lord Jesus Christ.*
>
> *In the representative and substitutionary sacrificial death of our Lord Jesus Christ as the necessary atonement for our sins.*
>
> *In the presence and power of the Holy Spirit in the work of regeneration. In the resurrection of the crucified body of our Lord, and that blessed hope, His personal return.*

As national interest in CMS grew, the first one-page edition of the "CMS News" rolled off a borrowed mimeograph machine on January 1, 1941, in an attempt to communicate the vision more broadly. It read, in part:

> *Doctor....we would like to introduce ourselves with this paper. We are sending it to you because you are a Christian as well as a doctor; we believe that you are interested in other Christians in the same profession and in things that they are doing....*

The newsletter also included this ad:

Sending out that newsletter was a step of faith. The publication continued to use the Fourth Presbyterian Church's mimeograph machine until the group acquired a used hand-fed one, which was moved into the research lab. The newsletter was edited and printed in after-school hours. But there was also a need for a small stencil duplicator for printing postcards. One day Joe Boutwell was in one of Chicago's large stationery stores inquiring about such a machine when another customer asked about his interest in the duplicator. When Joe told him of CMS, the stranger reached in his pocket and said, "Here, let me help," and paid the clerk. CMS never learned the identity of the benefactor, which gave a deeper meaning to a headline in the next newsletter: "Strange—Yet Not So Strange for Those Who Trust."

The July 1942 "CMS News," a mimeographed newsletter, announced the acceptance of the Christian Medical Society of Greater New York as the second chapter in the national organization. The Executive Committee pro tem had earlier accepted the Chicago Society—Northwestern and the University of Illinois combined—as the first local chapter.

The emphasis remained on reaching medical students. "Feeler" letters were sent to schools around the country. Other chapters which joined in the early '40s included Jefferson Medical School and the Women's Medical College in Philadelphia, and others in Albany, Minnesota, and Oregon. By the middle 40s the Philadelphia student work was thriving with chapters in all five medical schools.

Under the leadership of the president of the Chicago organization, Dr. John D. Frame, Jr. (later a missionary to Iran and a tropical medicine specialist as an Associate Professor of Public Health at Columbia University), the Society took the important step of the formation of a national organization during the 1941-42 year. The new constitution called for an Executive Committee of five members to carry out the policies of CMS. The Executive Committee was made up of those from the Chicago area until the organization might become large enough and members could afford to travel to take part in leadership deci-

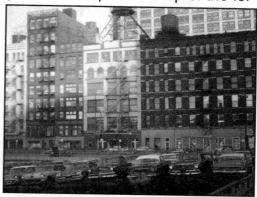

The CMS office was located in the tallest of the buildings shown here at 64 W. Randolph Street.

sion-making. The "CMS News" progressed to four pages of real print in 1945.

In 1946, the certificate of incorporation was granted by the state of Illinois. The first president of the new national organization was a medical student at the University of Illinois, James Krafft, an editor of the single-sheet "CMS News." His wife was then the office secretary. Dr. Krafft recalls his election:

> The tremendous presence of Kenneth Gieser in those days was our inspiration. But I think about that time he had gone to do eye work at Kano, Nigeria, for one of his six-month visits. There was the need for a national president. I don't remember the details, but I think Jonathan Cilley and Joe Boutwell felt that the first president of the national CMS should be a medical student. I think they probably called Del Nelson and a couple of others over in the University of Illinois and said, "We ought to make Jim president." I think it was a major vote of about five or six! So I became president in 1946, but the records show I became a member in 1947!

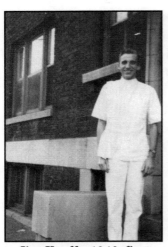

Jim Krafft, 1946, first CMS president, as a medical student.

CMS had begun as a work with students. Dr. Bill Johnson recalled, "As a medical student, I was a three-year-old Christian when I went, and to find a group of friends who loved the Lord and were ready to serve Him was such a blessing to me. I found medical school a very turbulent time. I had the desire to witness to my buddies that I sat next to in the lab, but I found it hard."

As the students were moving on after training, more interest in CMS was gradually growing among graduate physicians, and notices appeared in the "CMS News" listing opportunities to practice here and abroad.

To help CMS members better fulfill their sense of calling to witness to their peers, *Quote...Unquote*, the first venture of CMS-published resources, carried personal testimonies of faith by ten physicians who had attained recognition in their respective fields at that time, including: Howard A. Kelly, M.D., Professor Emeritus of Gynecology, Johns Hopkins University; William A. MacPherson, M.D., Captain, U.S. Army Medical Corps; Paul E. Adolph, M.D., Missionary to China; J. Paul Bennett, M.D.,

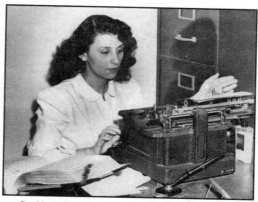

Sally Krafft served as the first CMS secretary for her husband, Dr. Jim Krafft.

Instructor of Roentgenology, Cook County Graduate School of Medicine; John R. Brobeck, M.D., Assistant Professor of Physiology, Yale University Medical School; William H. Chisholm, M.D., Medical Missionary to Korea; Thomas M. Durant, M.D., Associate Professor of Internal Medicine, Temple University; Bruce V. MacFadyen, M.D., Clinical Professor of Gynecology, Hahneman Medical College; Cecil P. Martin, M.B., Sc.D., Professor of Anatomy, McGill University; Everett D. Sugarbaker, M.D., Chief Surgeon & Medical Director, Ellis Fischel State Cancer Hospital, Missouri.

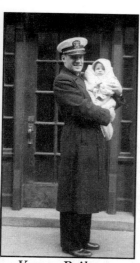

Vernoy Reihmer, M.D., CMS President, 1947.

The cost for printing the two editions of *Quote...Unquote* (totaling 20,000 copies) was covered by a generous gift from Dr. Cilley's father in law, Robert E. Nicholas, as the small weekly offerings of the medical students—many working their way through school—were not large enough to afford such an undertaking. Besides being made available to CMS members for their own evangelistic use, the booklet was mailed to every physician listed in the yellow pages.

Missions took a prominent place in the "CMS News" with exciting reports from the growing number of members now serving around the world as their vision had widened after World

War II. But as an article in April 1947 said, the cost of becoming a medical missionary was considerable:

A nationally known drug company recently stated in one of its advertisements that it takes eight years of hard study and an investment of about $15,000 before a doctor is ready to practice. It would seem important, therefore, for a servant of the Lord to have a fairly clear idea how he intends to use his life on the mission field before he invests such a staggering amount of time, effort, and money.

The World War II years brought new emphasis in the "CMS News." Prayer requests were included from those in the armed forces scattered around the world, leading Bible study classes and prayer meetings aboard ship or in camp. Notices of those killed in action were also printed. **Ophthalmologist** Dr. William MacPherson had shared his testimony in *Quote....Unquote*: "I believe that Jesus Christ bore the guilt of my sin as He suffered on the cross. Acceptance of Him as Lord and Savior **opened my blind eyes**, so

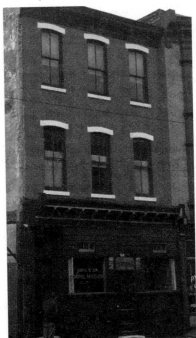

that now thanks to Him, *I may see the glories of God's spiritual world, **both here and hereafter**"* (editor's emphasis). He was killed in action in Okinawa in 1945.

Dr. Oliver Austin was often mentioned in the early news. As a student at Northwestern, he had been burdened to reach his fellow students. "I am planning to go to the mission field, but I may never get there," he said. "My life work may be going to medical school. The time to serve the Lord is now." He led the Chicago society in 1940 in expansion to students. But he never did get to the mission field. As he was serving in the United States Army Medical Corps, orders sent him to an obscure post in northern Canada. On his last mercy flight to an Indian village with a serious

Site of "John 5:24" Mission, another Philadelphia mission clinic.

14

epidemic of septic sore throat, his small plane crashed into Hudson Bay in 1945. His Army associates noted that he was "more than an excellent surgeon...a true follower of Christ."

With CMS growing, it was time to move the national headquarters out of the cramped alcove in the corner of the Northwestern lab. In 1945 Drs. Cilley and Boutwell found a place at 189 West Madison Street in the heart of Chicago, and they moved into a twelve-by-seventeen-foot room on the ninth floor. They paid $45 a month, and purchased used furniture. A metal file cabinet, however, was put on hold because of lack of funds. After years of office help from the wives of members, CMS hired its first full-time—and paid—secretary. The new monthly budget for the entire CMS operation was $215, and members were urged to adopt a plan of systematic giving toward this.

Before long there were more moves. The end of 1946 brought a new office home at 64 East Lake Street with proximity to other Christian organizations headquartered in the building. But by the end of the decade CMS was unable to meet a rent increase, so another transfer was made, this time to 64 West Randolph Street, still in downtown Chicago. InterVarsity Christian Fellowship (InterVarsity) was housed there and they offered a choice of offices in the suite they were leasing, which provided much needed additional space.

As a close relationship developed between InterVarsity and CMS, InterVarsity (which works mostly on student campuses) invited CMS to join them. But CMS did not wish to remain just a student group. Its leaders looked forward to the years when CMS would also be a graduate organization, maintaining a specific focus for the medical profession. In 1947 the "CMS News" said, "The society is becoming an organization led by physicians, with a decrease in the burden of work carried by medical students. This is as it should be, and has been the ultimate aim of the organization since its conception."

The time had also come to consider a National Convention. The first—where sixty-four gathered, thirty-three from outside Chicago—was held at the Chicago Illini Union Building in June 1947. A second followed there in 1948. In 1949 the convention was held in Philadelphia. Travel was a challenge, and Dr. John Elsen (President,

1948) recalls, "It was quite a trip—no expressways at that time. The car was full and we drove all night from Chicago, up and down Route 40. But I remember the warm reception." National conventions continued until 1956, meeting in Chicago, Philadelphia, New York, San Francisco, and Atlantic City. Often the conventions were at the same place as the AMA annual meeting, since many CMS doctors would already be traveling there.

At early CMS conventions, psychiatry subjects attracted much attention. Articles related to psychiatry appeared regularly in the "CMS News." CMS wanted to make an impact on theory and practice in the field of psychiatry. In 1947 Dr. John Hyde, a pediatric allergist, was the first to head the CMS "psychiatry section," and for years Dr. William H. Whitely, a neurosurgeon, was the psychiatric editor of the CMS publications until psychiatrists became interested in CMS. The psychiatry section was officially formed and recognized by CMS in 1964 and has remained active through the years.

Following the war, the missionary membership continued to grow as letters came from every mission field. The war had taken members overseas and their vision had increased. The idea for "The League of Brother Physicians" came in 1949 from the young CMS chapter in New Orleans. They suggested that physicians "adopt" a medical missionary. As the stateside doctors became acquainted with their brother physicians' needs and problems on the field, they would be able to help in practical ways—sending medical texts and literature, aiding in purchasing, making ham radio contact, and supporting them in prayer. In the '50s this came under the umbrella of the Medical Missionary Fellowship in CMS.

There was a mission attitude locally, too. One Sunday evening in 1948 a medical student at the University of Pennsylvania, H. Newton Spencer, had a date with a medical technician whose father was going to a service at the Central Gospel Hall Mission in Philadelphia. He invited his daughter and her date to go with him. Sitting on the platform, the medical student looked out on the sea of faces of some seven hundred fifty men and women whose bodies and souls appeared broken. Straining to hear the preaching of

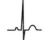

16

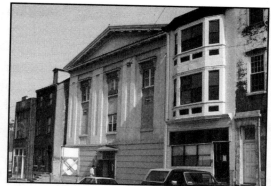

Central Gospel Hall in Philadelphia (the columned building) was the site of the first CMS mission clinic.

Christ in a room saturated with coughs and groans, he asked himself: *Why not establish a medical mission right here?*

The directors of the Central Gospel Hall Mission and the Eighth Street Wayside Mission agreed that a medical clinic would meet a dire need. A room was immediately made available and physicians donated equipment and supplies. But when permission was sought from the medical school for students to serve at the mission, there was concern that the majority of the personnel would not have licenses to practice medicine. So the project was renamed "Medical Counseling Service" by the University of Pennsylvania. Permission was granted for the students to do anything that a visiting nurse or druggist could legally do. The Philadelphia County Medical Society granted their wholehearted support, and permission was also given for students from any of the five medical schools in Philadelphia to participate.

The first mission "clinic" opened in March 1949. The first patients to arrive were just two sick and curious men. The next week there were four. Soon, however, word spread about the kind care, and the benches were filled every Sunday. "John 5:24 Mission" joined the two other mission clinics, and students continued to work under the supervision of Dr. Kenneth Scott, a resident in surgery who later served as a Presbyterian medical missionary in Korea, followed by years as principal of the Ludiana Medical College in India. The University of Pennsylvania required that a faculty member supervise, and prayers were answered when Dr. C. Everett Koop, then Chief of Surgery at the Children's Hospital, became active in CMS and then became the director.

A similar scenario resulted in the establishment of the CMS mission clinic at the Pacific Garden Mission in Chicago in 1950. "I prayed for ten years for a medical clinic," said Harry Saulnier, mission superintendent. "Then one day Dean Smith, a University of Illinois medical student, and two fellow students came to the mission. They timidly asked if they might start a clinic." Once the clinic was established, it continued there for years.

The mission clinics began with motivation from students, but graduate members also became enthusiastic about helping in these clinics. It was felt that it was necessary to have at least one licensed physician as a sponsor for each clinic. Graduates could not always find time for CMS graduate meetings, but they liked the practical

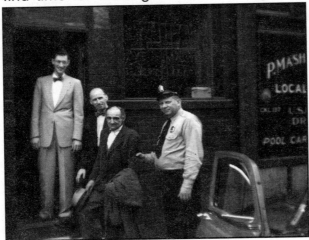

ministry. Mission clinics were established around the country in needy areas of cities—by 1955 there were twelve.

Toward the end of the 1940s, the Executive Committee realized the need to share more of the leadership in the organization of CMS. In 1949 it was agreed that there be a Board of

"John 5:24" Mission Clinic:
Your choice. Clinic or jail?

Directors including physicians—elected for three years—and students—elected for one year. The Board would then choose its Executive Committee of six physicians and two students from the Chicago area, convenient to the central office.

Gradually there had come interest from some dentists who had heard of this Christian professional organization. There was talk that a separate Christian dental society might be formed outside of CMS, but a news note in a 1945 "CMS News" welcomed dentists. It seems that for some years they were considered associate members, but the revised 1950 constitution specified that they were to be full members.

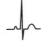

CMS was growing. Graduate chapters were being formed all around the country, most in the eastern half, and there was much that needed to be done to encourage the new groups. Dr. Bill Johnson recalls that during his internship and residency days he, and others like him, did brief field director-like stints to visit chapters in the Midwest and East.

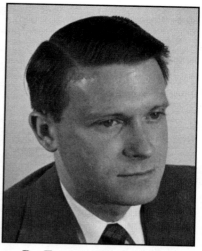

Dr. Emmett Herring, first Executive Secretary.

At the second annual convention in Chicago in 1948, CMS President Dr. John Elsen announced that God had answered the prayers of many for the need of an Executive Secretary, someone who would travel around the country to make contacts. Dr. Emmett Herring, who was completing internship at Charity Hospital in New Orleans, was the man appointed. Dr. Elsen said that the monthly salary and travel expense budget totaled $350 per month, a financial burden he acknowledged, but that they would move ahead by faith. He quoted an executive committee member, "If this were a worldly organization, I would say that taking on the responsibility of an executive secretary would be impossible and ridiculous, but with God all things are possible."

Dr. Herring was no stranger to the Chicago group as he had transferred to the University of Illinois Medical School from Mississippi for his junior year, and had been very active in CMS. The late Dr. Herring, when a retired ophthalmologist in Mississippi, recalled those days as Executive Secretary: "I traveled by bus from coast to coast. I stayed in the homes of members to cut costs, and in my briefcase I carried an extra set of wash-and-wear underwear. I washed the day's wear each evening in a CMS member's home." While Emmett considered the Elsens' a place to leave his things, Dr. Elsen says, "He didn't even have a room; he just traveled."

Dr. Johnson recalls the sacrifice Emmett made, "Those were the days when residencies were hard fought for with everyone coming back from the service, so it was highly competitive. So I feel Emmett

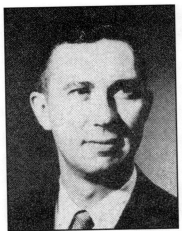

really felt called of the Lord to do this even at the risk of not getting a residency."

Dr. Herring served for two years with CMS before going to serve in the Armed Forces during the Korean War. He was God's appointed man to encourage the growth of CMS as he traveled throughout the country, meeting with students, recruiting graduates, training leadership, and making others aware of the national scope of CMS.

Dr. William Johnson, the first editor of the new Journal

There was an increased sense that CMS needed someone to continue to do the job which Emmett had begun, laying the groundwork well for another Executive Secretary to come.

During the 1940s, as a result of an expanding vision and quality leadership, CMS continued to grow. By 1949, the number of local chapters, nationwide, was twenty-five. Student groups were meeting on many campuses. In 1949, the "CMS News" became the well-designed *Christian Medical Society Journal*, published quarterly. Dr. William A. Johnson (CMS president, 1960-61) was the *Journal's* first editor.

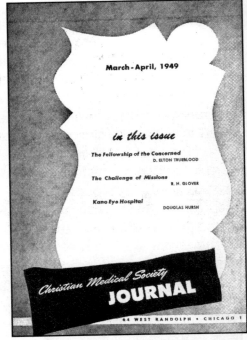

March-April, 1949

in this issue

The Fellowship of the Concerned
D. ELTON TRUEBLOOD

The Challenge of Missions
R. H. GLOVER

Kano Eye Hospital
DOUGLAS HURSH

Christian Medical Society JOURNAL

44 WEST RANDOLPH • CHICAGO 1

The first issue of the CMS Journal (March - April 1949)

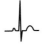

Chapter 3

The Building Years with Mission Emphasis: The 1950s

*I*n 1951 the President of CMS, Dr. Howard Hamlin, came back to Chicago from a CMS convention in Philadelphia, intent on putting the CMS office in order. The office had actually been closed for awhile because of staff problems. Dr. Hamlin, a surgeon who was still doing some general practice at that time, took time one September morning to make a house call. A family from his church had two sick children. He went to an apartment in the old house next to the church, where Ray and Beth Knighton lived with their family.

Dr. Hamlin's heart was heavy with the needs of CMS. He shared with Ray how CMS desperately needed someone to fill the position of Executive Secretary since Emmett Herring's departure. He looked at Ray Knighton and said, "Ray, you've done some administrative work when you were teaching. Why don't you come and run CMS?"

Ray Knighton had taught at a Nazarene college in Idaho, but now he was working on his Ph.D. in music in Chicago. He had expected to teach that September at the Chicago Evangelistic Institute while working on this degree, but had just learned that the school was moving to Iowa.

"I was without a job, and Howard knew that," Ray recalled. "I wasn't that interested in his offer, but he convinced me to go with him to an executive committee meeting at Dr. Paul Adolph's home in Wheaton."

J. Raymond Knighton, Jr., the new Executive Secretary (1951)

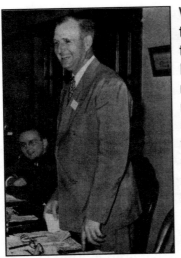

Dr. H. Hamlin,
President 1951, at
convention banquet.

When the board asked Knighton to take the position in October, it was only part-time because CMS could afford no more. Ray agreed to help CMS out for a couple of months, for which he was paid $75 a month. There was no contract, according to Ray, "...just an agreement with the Lord that I would serve Him." But as Ray saw the vision and became so engrossed in the work of CMS, this soon became full-time, and his music became a part-time ministry.

Dr. Ralph Blocksma recalled the financial struggles of the Society in those years. "At one point we didn't have enough money to keep Ray in groceries even on his pathetic salary, so a special appeal to the known membership was made to chip in and save the Society. They did. Ray's wife, Beth, continued to play the organ for funerals to make ends meet, but they never threw in the sponge."

A man of vision and energy, with the warmth of an outgoing personality always reaching out to others, Knighton brought a tremendous surge to the growth of the Society. He took CMS "...to dizzying heights," according to a past president, Dr. Bill Johnson. Through the fourteen years that Ray Knighton served as Executive Secretary (a position that was later called General Director) of CMS, he was often recognized as "Mr. CMS."

Ray continued to travel around the country visiting medical campuses and graduate chapters, while at the same time overseeing the growing office work and editing the *Journal*. But Ray needed to be two people at least in order to get everything done. The urgent prayer request for CMS was for a director of student work. This prayer was answered with the coming of Bill Ramer. Bill, an InterVarsity staff member, was introduced to the Society when he hosted the CMS group at InterVarsity's Bear Trap Ranch for one of CMS's earliest family conferences. During the next year it became evident to both organizations that Bill should work among the medical students, so he became affiliated with CMS in 1955.

The student work continued to flourish, and Bill Ramer needed help. At the same time the CMS leaders were praying about this, a young doctor across the Atlantic in Denmark was asking the Lord to lead him to a place to serve during his upcoming one-year visit to the States. C. Stacey Woods, General Secretary of InterVarsity, met Dr. Vagh Brondum during a tour of Denmark, and asked him, "Have you heard of the Christian Medical Society?" Although Dr. Brondum had not heard of CMS, he was very interested, and the doors opened for him to help Bill Ramer for a year.

The Society's emphasis remained on students. The work continued to grow and another student staff member—Stanley Bigelow—was added to the staff in 1958. Bigelow came with seminary training and background as an assistant pastor. This was just the beginning of growth of a field staff, where many have served through the years.

Attempts at regional conferences for students met with varying success. The first national student conference, focused on the theme of campus evangelism and held in September 1955 in Des Plaines, Illinois, was attended by thirty students. Out of that gathering came a strong demand for more such conferences, which have continued through the years.

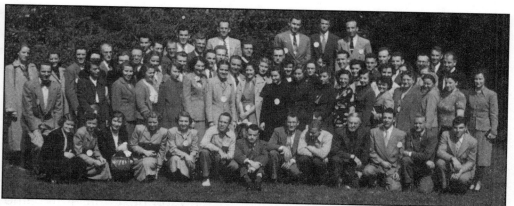

First Regional Conference (1950) at Bethana, Pa.

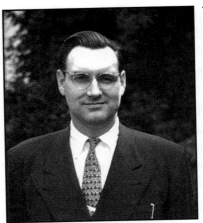

Dr. C. Everett Koop, Regional Conference Speaker, then Chief of Surgery at Children's Hospital in Pa.

The medical families also had needs. Ray Knighton now sees the development of family conferences as one of the most important projects to have been started in the '50s. He recalls that he was approached by Sam Fuenning who said, "Ray, there has to be a place where doctors and their families can go and enjoy fellowship, talk shop, and get to know one another."

"So we arranged to go to Bear Trap Ranch, an InterVarsity camp outside of Colorado Springs, for a week in the summer of 1952," Ray said. "The camp was in pitiful shape. The only way to get to it was to drive up what used to be a railroad grade with the ties still in. There was nothing for the kids to do—no swimming pool or any other recreational facility. Beth ran a vacation Bible school.

"Well, in spite of our rocky start, family conferences never stopped," Knighton added. "The next two years we used Young Life's Silver Cliff Camp. It was there we met someone who had bought the land right next to that camp and had started Deer Valley Ranch. We went there in 1955, and CMDA is still going there for family conferences today." Other places have also hosted camps through the years, but Deer Valley Ranch remains a favorite.

Life-changing decisions are made at these conferences. Ray recalled from the early days, "Every Friday night we had a sharing time before leaving on Saturday morning. One such night when we were sitting in front of the fireplace I noticed that Wally and Charlotte Swanson, who were from Minneapolis, were there. They had stayed in the lodge right next to us, but we hadn't seen much of them all week. Wally hadn't even come to meals.

"Finally, when we were there in our sharing time, Wally got up and started pacing back and forth. He said, 'I've been wrestling with the Lord all week about the mission field. The Lord used this time here

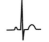

at Deer Valley to convince me that this is what we should do.' Wally took up most of the rest of the evening just sharing how the Lord was leading him and his wife to go into missionary medicine at the HCJB Hospital in Quito, Ecuador, where he served for many years."

But doctors also began to notice another mission opportunity right in their "back yards," as an increasing number of foreign physicians took advanced training in the United States. Noting that many of them would be the future leaders in their own countries, CMS doctors saw this as a mission field. They could invite these international doctors into their homes and build friendships with them.

One of those who was reached through this friendship evangelism was Tai Joon Moon, M.D., from Korea. Four years after he had returned to Korea to practice neurosurgery in Seoul, Dr. Moon's story appeared in the April-May-June 1958 CMS Journal, excerpted here:

> When I walked into the Neurosurgical Department of Jefferson Hospital in Philadelphia, I was very eager to learn the advanced knowledge and technique for the needy peoples of my fatherland, but I felt emptiness in a corner of my heart, which had many unhappy scars. I was born into a Buddhist family but had very little contact with Buddhism. During my school days I was compelled to worship at the Shinto-shrine, but I felt no response in my heart. Then, at the end of World War II came liberation of our country from foreign domination, and I suddenly had to face the rapid social changes and the two entirely different ways of thinking: democracy and communism. Through the terrible war I experienced many distressing things which made me have a very dim view of human life. The changes in scenery and way of living in the United States failed to erase these scars.
>
> My life as a resident in Jefferson Hospital in Philadelphia was very pleasant and profitable. As time passed, however, and the end of my stay was drawing near, I began to realize that something very important was lacking in myself. The Lord made me find the answer by showing me three important factors: 1) He gave me an opportunity to work under one of the best Christians I have met. This surgeon [Dr. William

Whiteley—a past president of CMS] showed me the true meaning of the Christian life through his acts in addition to his talk; 2) Through my daily work in the hospital the Lord made me realize that the patients were in need of help spiritually as well as physically. Not being born again, I was of no use to them beyond a certain extent; and, 3) The Lord showed me two different types of patients. When they were told about the incurable diseases they had, one group showed mental bankruptcy. True Christians kept peace of mind because they left themselves in God's will and desire.

Dr. Moon went on to say, "I often wondered how I could believe things I could not explain. But I finally made the decision and accepted Jesus Christ as my Savior. Life has different meaning now."

The graduate chapters were also increasing throughout the United States and the fellowship dinners at the AMA and specialty meetings were important. The doctors talked more and more about their

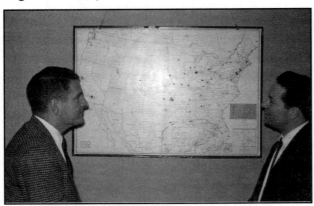

Bill Ramer (l.) Stanley Bigelow (r.), two field staff, look at map with 60 pins representing student chapters

responsibility to mentor students and not just to emphasize their fellowship with one another.

Medical evangelism became more evident in these years, and CMS saw what was considered an unusual opportunity to present Christ to the medical profession during the AMA's annual meeting in San Francisco in 1958. Billy Graham was to be in town for a campaign, and the Society invited all of the officers of the AMA, plus many other leading medical people, to attend a luncheon, as guests of CMS, to hear Billy Graham speak. More than 400 people were present, even though it was the first day of the annual meeting, with little time for advance publicity of this special event.

This decade saw an explosion in the missionary movement. In the 1950s the ratio of missionary doctors in the membership was high, about a fourth of the membership. Ray Knighton kept in close contact with them. The CMS "News and Reports" (a regular newsletter published for years in addition to the *Journal)* listed many missionary visitors to the CMS office. It was a good place to stop by and the Chicago area was convenient for travel through the country.

"We were constantly helping CMS members who were planning to go the mission field," Ray Knighton remembers. "We started doing some general purchasing for them, getting good discounts because of their work. Then when they got to the field, many of them wrote with urgent requests for help in finding drugs and supplies. Or sometimes it was for treatment advice, and I found CMS doctors who could give the right information."

Not finding any organization to help address these needs, Knighton began to make his own contacts with drug and medical supply companies. These companies respected the work of the missionary physicians, and the lists of needs grew longer. Then one day in April 1954 Ray got a call from Art Larsen in the advertising division of Scherring Company. He said, "I just shipped you eleven tons of drugs worth $26,000."

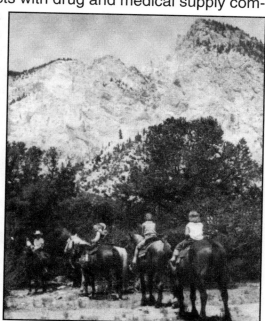

Ray's shocked reaction was, "You did what? How did you know about us?" Larsen explained that every Monday night he attended Dr. Donald Grey Barnhouse's Bible study in New York City. When Larsen told him about his company's

Families began enjoying trips to Deer Valley Ranch in Nathrop, Co.

need to get rid of a surplus of good medical pharmaceuticals, Dr. Barnhouse had replied, "Oh, I know a big guy who knows every

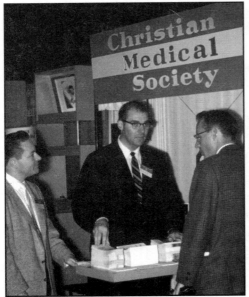
The first CMS booth at the 1959 AMA Convention

medical missionary in the world—send them to him!"

Larsen had the impression that Ray was all set up with a warehouse. Had Larsen contacted Ray prior to sending the shipment, Ray says he would have turned it down. But according to Ray, "When the trucking dispatcher called and asked, 'Where do you want me to put this stuff?' I said, '108 North Dearborn!'" This was in the middle of Chicago, where CMS had moved its offices in 1952.

The next day when the semi pulled up (semis usually didn't come to that area) Ray went to the stationery store across the street and bought a small cart to move the stuff. He describes the ordeal, "There was no freight elevator in the building, so I had to unload this semi about four cases at a time up the passenger elevator to the fifth floor. It took me all day.

"We didn't have any other place to put it," he said, "so we put it in the small office, about thirty feet square. We were a staff of only four—three women and myself. I piled the boxes at the edge of the room, afraid to put them in the middle because the building wasn't that sturdy! About three weeks later some space opened up in another part of the building.

"The AMA annual convention was in Chicago in June, so I let all the missionary doctors on furlough within a 500-mile radius know of this. I got on

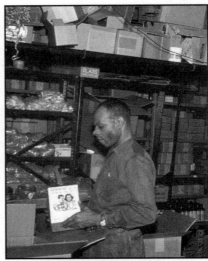
The original MAP warehouse

the phone and said, 'Look, we have all this medicine. Bring a trailer or station wagon and get this out of here!'" Most of the stuff was gone after the AMA meeting, so Ray didn't need to ship anything!

This new venture for CMS became known as the Missionary Assistance Program, later called MAP International (the Medical Assistance Program).

The unsolicited receipt of donations from drug and supply companies increased rapidly. These companies felt they could give to CMS with confidence that their surpluses would be properly distributed to trusted missionary physicians. The lists of donations included such useful drugs such as terramycin, penicillin, and streptomycin, but one list of donations even included 19,500 sets of posterior porcelain teeth!

A big concern was the lack of space for this growing ministry to missionaries. In early 1957, with nine employees now at the office, the Society moved from North Dearborn to 127 South Wacker Drive, where there was more room and proximity to major transportation facilities. And…there was a freight elevator! This building was owned by a Christian foundation, which welcomed Christian organizations.

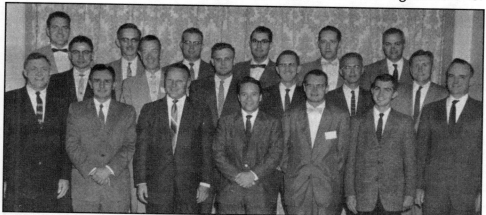

The CMS 1958 Board of Directors with CMS Presidents noted in bold
(l. to r.): D. Nelson M.D., K. Gieser M.D., J. Young M.D., S. Bigelow,
J. Hyde M.D., K. Zwagerman, W. Erdman M.D.
2nd Row: R. Schiedt (medical student), G. Hemwall M.D.,
P. Jorden M.D., R. Blocksma M.D., W. Whiteley M.D.
3rd Row: B. Ramer, J. Frame M.D., D. Busby M.D., R. Knighton,
E. Van Reken M.D., R. Gottlieb M.D.
(Editor's note: Listing of all Presidents with dates in the appendix)

Knighton also began to hear medical missionaries ask for a different kind of help. They asked if doctors couldn't come even for a short visit to help them. To address this need, during this decade CMS developed a new mission strategy, a forerunner of the short-term missions concept which mission organizations were not ready to consider at that time. The goal was to connect members interested in helping medical missionaries for short periods of time with missionaries who had expressed the need for help. The Christian Medical Society Foundation was formed to assist in arranging these visits.

Plastic surgeon Dr. Ralph Blocksma (a past president) and his wife, Ruth, were among the first to participate in this new program. They had been missionaries in Pakistan but had returned because of Ralph's health. Now, through the CMS short-term missions, they

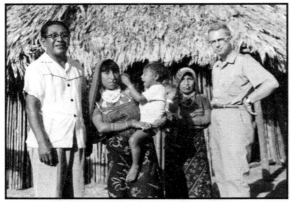

Dr. Ralph Blocksma, plastic surgeon, on mission tirp to San Blas Islands

found themselves going to a number of different countries. Dr. Blocksma called it "tithing for Christ," giving of his time to go where a plastic surgeon was so needed.

With the high interest in medical missions during those years, could more networking be done? There were missionary conferences, but were there specific tracks for medical missions? CMS sensed a need. So near the end of this decade, between Christmas and New Year's 1959, the first International Convention on Missionary Medicine (ICMM) sponsored by CMS was held at Wheaton College in Illinois.

Far exceeding the expectation of its planners, this event brought together more than 750 furloughing missionary physicians, prospective medical missionaries, residents and interns, nurses, mission board executives, and others interested in medical missionary work.

Delegates came from thirty-nine U.S. states, four Canadian provinces, and twenty-five foreign countries. Missionaries and mission executives represented forty-five boards. The attendance grew to 1,200 for evening meetings open to the public.

The speakers' roster included such well-known leaders as A.W. Tozer, Drs. L. Nelson Bell, Ralph Blocksma, Robert Cochrane, then CMS President P. Kenneth Gieser, and C. Everett Koop. This event was met with such enthusiasm that similar conven-

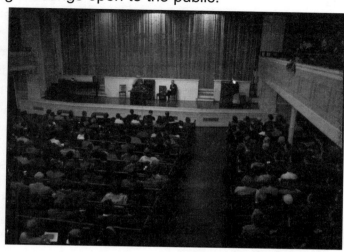

"The Man God Uses" was the theme of the 1959 ICMM Conference held at Wheaton College.

tions were scheduled biennially until the mid '60s, continuing later under the work of MAP International.

The decade of the '50s brought expansion of student work, growth of graduate fellowships with purposeful outreach, addition of family conferences, and an explosion of medical mission interest. The Christian Medical Society was building characteristics in the organization that would last through the years.

Dr. Delbert Nelson (CMS President, 1957-58) recalled that there were some tough times, too, often related to funding. But, he said, "We were making progress."

Chapter 4

Multiplication And Division:
The 1960s

*B*y 1960, the growth of CMS demanded more space than was available at Wacker Drive in Chicago. Since the cost of rent in the city was out of reach for anything larger, the organization's leaders began looking nearby for a building that would offer better long-term possibilities.

Mr. Robert Nicholas, father of an active CMS member Dr. Everett Nicholas, was instrumental in finding a two-story building, approximately thirty years old, in excellent condition, located in nearby Oak Park, Illinois. The elderly couple who owned the building graciously accepted an annuity-type payment arrangement for the building, which was deeded to CMS in 1960.

A warehouse for the increasing donations of medical equipment, drugs and supplies for CMS's Medical Assistance Program (MAP) was found in Forest Park, just one and a half blocks from the new CMS headquarters. This building's three floors were already bulging soon after the move, as the "News and Reports" said, "...with everything from toothpaste to second-hand sterilizers."

In 1960 the Field Department was formed. Stanley Bigelow had already been serving as a Student Secretary, but now he consented to serve as Field Secretary for the union of student work and the emerging ministry among practicing doctors. New field men were Dr. Charles Crown, who with his general practice in the Chicago area, would

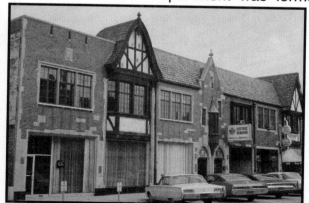

CMS Headquarters in Oak Park, Illinois

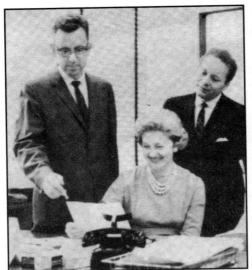

Field Dept. formed 1960. (l. to r.)
Dr. Charles Crown, Field Staff;
Rachael Buick, Secretary; Stanley
Bigelow, Field Director.

work on a part-time basis for two years, and John Lepp.

For these new CMS field staff members, there was the usual pressure of travel, and many contacts made to encourage the growing number of student and graduate chapters. But in order to bring more members together for fellowship, a lot of energy went into arranging regional CMS conferences throughout the country—twelve of these occurring in the fall of 1961.

As the ministry grew, new staffing strategies developed. In 1962, a decision was reached that leadership was to come from regional staff placed in specific geographical areas, working on the grassroots level. The first regional staff member was a Texan with theological training, Robert Metzger. A few months later Dr. Mel Alexander, a psychologist from California, came on board. Eight regions were envisioned initially, but Metzger and Alexander could only cover two each, leaving the rest vacant for the time being.

In 1964, another field staff member was hired to cover the region of the Northeastern United States and Eastern Canada. Lewis Bird, S.T.M. (who later earned a Ph.D.) had just finished his work on a master's degree in Theology at Chicago Lutheran Seminary while serving in a church in the area. He had become familiar with CMS and welcomed the opportunity. Lew served CMS until his retirement in 1996. At the 1997 National Conference, Lew was presented with an honorary membership by incoming president Dr. Dorothy Barbo. A tribute to Dr. Bird, published in the Winter 1996 issue of *Today's Christian Doctor*, said, "With an infectious wit and tireless dedication, Lew sought to bring serious biblical reflection to bioethical dilemmas and a pastor's heart to the personal pain of student and doctor alike." Former President Dr. Robert Scheidt said, "We have explored friendship's high country together—literally at the Colorado Mining town, and figuratively when we tried for Jesus' sake to wrestle with the moral issues confronting Christian doctors in our society…. You once wrote a compliment to me…(that) I now return to you. 'Heaven will be Lew Bird living around the corner.'"

Another field man who served CMS for years was Sid Macaulay, Th.M. He came from a pastorate in Virginia to be the Southeastern Regional Representative in 1968, serving until 1991 when he died from a sudden heart attack. Former General Director Hal Habecker, D. Min., said, "Sid poured his life into his regional ministry. He loved students and doctors, and he loved encouraging them. He was always enthusiastic…always thinking ahead." Lew Bird eulogized Sid at his memorial service, "Sid was my friend. He was my friend and colleague for twenty-four years. We roomed together, we shaved together, we laughed together, we prayed together, we deliberated together, we jogged together, we hiked together, we sailed together. Sid died on my birthday. I turned fifty-eight, and he entered a new year by entering a new life."

Sid was remembered for his work in editing the *Journal* as well. Dr. John Brobeck said, "Comparing Christian publications, I believe our *Journal* is one of the best. Sid was an excellent editor, with very good judgment and a knack for editing. I don't know how he did it combined with his regional responsibilities."

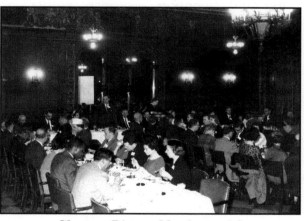

Chapter Dinner Meetings with special speakers were important.

By the end of the decade, six regions were covered. The additional staff included Haddon Robinson, Th.D. (South Central), Carl Saylor, (Midwest and North Central), Lynn Buzzard (Northwest), and Joseph Ludders, M.A. (Western Region). "Members in the western region remember Joe as industrious and verbally challenging," says regional director Michael McLaughlin, M.Div. "Often his postcards required a dictionary to decipher his meaning. But this extra work was always entertaining, and Joe and Kathy were much loved as Joe covered a territory from the western border of Texas to Alaska to Hawaii—and everything in between—for most of his nearly twenty years with the organization."

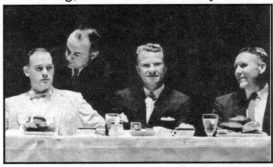

Breakfast with Billy Graham in Philadelphia; (l. to r.) Jay Ripka, student chairman; William Erdman, M.D.; Billy Graham; William H. Whitely, M.D., CMS President.

The field staff saw that leadership development was the key to effective student work. Lew and Sid organized the first Student Leadership Conference in 1969, when student chapter leaders came by invitation to Philadelphia. These conferences have continued, held now in each region once or twice a year, with a National Student Convention held concurrently with the National Convention.

There were other significant conferences in the decade. The First Latin America Congress, held at Quito, Ecuador in July 1964, was an outstanding success. This was a product of CMS's International Convention on Missionary Medicine as attendees felt that individual continental congresses would be valuable to address problems in specific locales. Both medical missionaries and nationals experienced a time of encouraging fellowship as well as exchange of viewpoints, even debate, but above all, promoting "the Kingdom of our Lord and Savior Jesus Christ in this world in our age."

In 1968, CMS told members that "A big Texas welcome awaits you!" The place was the "HemisFair '68" in San Antonio where representatives of thirty nations gathered to celebrate the 250th anniversary of the founding of San Antonio. CMS arranged a "Hemispheric Conference" at the same time as a creative witness. Internationally known physicians and speakers were a part of the program.

CMS-USA was helping its neighbors to the South by encouraging the establishment of a Christian Medical Society in Mexico. Two conventions were held there in the '60s. CMS-USA also assisted in planning the first Caribbean Convention of CMS in the Dominican Republic.

While things were moving ahead on the grassroots level, interest was building up for ministries overseas. Even the AMA hosted a Conference on Medical Missions, a historic one-day meeting with Christian medical mission leaders in August 1960 at the AMA headquarters. Ray Knighton took part in the discussion on how to assist medical missionary work.

By that time, the work of MAP within CMS was expanding rapidly. For Executive Director Ray Knighton this meant extensive travel overseas. In 1961 a call for help came from three physicians in the Congo–Drs. Warren and Gretchen Berggren and Dr. Glen Tuttle. The Belgian Congo had become independent and medical missionaries were badly in need of drugs and supplies. Knighton was instrumental in setting up the Congo Protestant Relief Agency, with other agencies cooperating. Ray was asked to survey the medical needs of ten countries in Africa. He was relieved to discover that two prominent physicians had also been asked to go—Drs. C. Everett Koop (then Professor of Surgery at the University of Pennsylvania) and Gus Hemwall (a past president and then a CMS board member).

During the five-week survey trip, the three visited medical establishments of twenty missionary societies, nine university and government hospitals, and six medical schools. Countries covered besides Congo were Egypt, Ethiopia, Kenya, Tanganyika, Uganda, Southern Rhodesia,

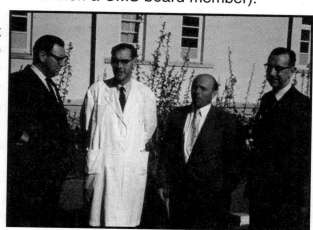

Dr. C. Everett Koop (l.) and Dr. Gus Hemwall (r.) on an assessment trip to Africa.

South Africa, Nigeria, and Ghana. The team traveled over 26,000 miles during this trip.

Ray came back increasingly challenged for MAP to help where it could. He also had developed a vision for the future of missionary medicine. In his report he said:

> Probably the greatest one area of the future medical mission-ary work is in the field of medical education. If the Church of Jesus Christ can train–not only competently qualified medical personnel–but also by precept and example show them that the greatest thing they can give to their people is the healing of the soul through believing and accepting Jesus Christ as Savior and Lord, we will have fulfilled our mission.

There still was much concern for the medical plight in Congo as doc-tors had fled the country during the Congolese fighting that followed independence, and medicine and supplies were all but impossible to procure. One young surgeon from California, who had joined CMS in 1954 while a student, answered the call to go on a short-term mis-sion trip in 1961 at the suggestion of Ray Knighton. Colleagues wrote, "The Congolese liked him immediately. He didn't complain about lack of facilities. There was a need, and he came to fill it. We thanked God for Paul Carlson."

A December 1964 CMS publication headline read: "CMS Member Dies in Congo." Dr. Paul Carlson had returned to Congo as a mis-sionary with the Evangelical Covenant Church of America. He had stayed at his hospital when others needed to be evacuated because of fighting. He was killed during the rebel massacre in Stanleyville on November 24, 1964. The colleagues who first asked for help in 1961 wrote: "We have no question about why Paul Carlson refused to desert his patients until he had to do so. Where there was a need, Paul did his utmost to fill it as he felt God led."

MAP had been known for the service of sending drugs and supplies to medical missionaries. But by 1964 this arm of CMS was offering more: educational services through conferences; short-term staff for mission hospitals through the Short Term Missionary Program; and, disaster relief projects—all of which required more organization and administrative support from the home office.

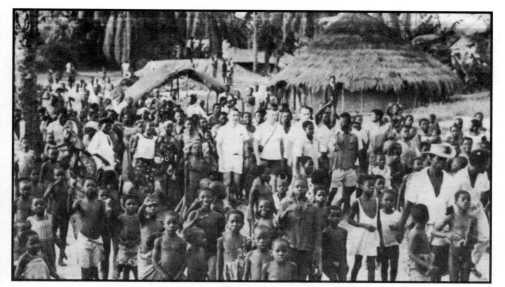

Dr. Carlson in the Congo (white shorts)

One relief project was in the Dominican Republic. In 1964 the Consul General of the Dominican Republic asked the president of CMS, Dr. Jim Krafft, if the Society would help establish infant rehydration centers as infants were dying at the rate of forty percent in the first year of life from dehydration due to dysentery. Knighton asked Dr. C. Everett Koop and Henry Harvey, a staff member, to go with him on an assessment trip. CMS and MAP then agreed to take on the challenge of establishing five infant rehydration centers throughout the country, with short-term workers staffing the facilities while MAP provided supplies. However, this project went so well that within the first three months, MAP had trained workers and set up units in twelve hospitals and the Ministry of Health was working in an additional twelve.

But there was another aspect of this Dominican project besides the children who were physically saved. Dr. Donald Johns, a pediatrician from Grand Rapids who went to help, saw this and wrote about it in the *Journal:*

Several Dominican doctors mentioned to me their gratitude and puzzlement over our willingness to help. This seemed to them a thankless and unremunerative mission. I had given scarcely thought about this aspect of the trip, having been trained to answer the call for medical assistance wherever I could best fit in. Yet it seems that when we exhibit simple loving concern without any ulterior motive, God, in His sovereignty, opens doors when we least expect it.

An experience I shared with one physician illustrates this. He asked me, one day, to tell him "the exact way." My thoughtless reply was that if he would follow me over to the wing of the hospital where the rehydration center was located, I would be happy to demonstrate it to him. His reply was, "Oh, no, I don't mean that. I want to know the way." I then went into a rather detailed explanation on how my wife had driven me to the airport where I had boarded the plane, and then told him of the route of the journey.

His patient answer was, "No, no, no, senor. Please, I wish to know the way to Christ whom you represent. I have heard something long ago about a straight and narrow way as well as the broad road. Perhaps you can tell me more?"

I had the opportunity to sit down with him ... and share God's simple invitation to men everywhere to come to Him by faith in His Son, Jesus Christ. This incident was typical of several during my stay in the Dominican Republic.

When CMS was introduced to the country via the national news media, physicians with Christian cnvictions began to make themselves publicly known. There is now a growing CMS there as a direct result of the rehydration program.

Dr. Martin Andrews, President of CMS in 1964-65, was one who went to help in the centers. But he also responded to another need when he was told about a four-year-old girl's serious congenital heart defect and her father's attempts to obtain treatment for her in the United States. Back in Oklahoma City, Dr. Andrews talked to heart surgeons who were willing to donate their services, and arrangements were made through ham radio contact to bring Ingrid and her parents, Mr. and Mrs. Vargas, there. Successful open-heart surgery followed, with no hospitalization charged at Deaconess Hospital. She and her grateful parents returned to Santo Domingo, leaving many friends in Oklahoma City who had been instrumental in Ingrid's care and her battle to gain the gift of life.

Things seemed to be expanding in all areas of the CMS work by the mid 1960s. But at the same time, there were concerns. Some were beginning to wonder if CMS was departing from her

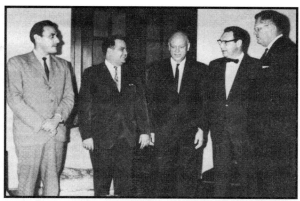

Dr. C Evertt Koop (second from r.) and MAP Director Henry Harvey (center) discuss rehydration project with Dominican Minister of Health (l.) and others.

first calling as a ministry to doctors and medical/dental students, and moving to an emphasis on a world-wide vision with the explosion of MAP's ministry. The question was, "What group or groups are we serving?"

There also was tension building between the Executive Director, Ray Knighton, and the Field Director, Stan Bigelow, with members involved with them starting to choose sides. The board made an unsuccessful effort to resolve the problems—which were partly philosophical, partly theological, and partly personal as in most such situations.

Thus, in November 1965 the CMS board voted to separate CMS and MAP. Some CMS board members immediately resigned and Dr. P. Kenneth Gieser, president of the board, stepped down as board president (while remaining a board member) to become president of the new MAP board.

MAP's initial board roster included thirteen CMS board members, some of whom continued to serve on the CMS board. Their first action was to employ Ray Knighton as Executive Director. The MAP office relocated in Glen Ellyn, without interruption of services.

The CMS publication "News and Reports" of January 1966 announced a "New Vision Developed for CMS and MAP." The article stated that the CMS board had authorized separate incorporation for MAP, and that "MAP's new framework will permit it to channel certain government services to medical missionaries abroad, and has created an organization with more possibilities for service than MAP has had in the past." It went on to say, "The CMS central organization, now somewhat smaller, is freer to clarify and implement its original vision as a fellowship for doctors and students with a positive Christian witness to colleagues."

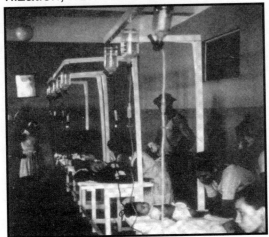
MAP rehydration centers set up in Dominican government hospitals

The next two years were spent trying to stabilize the Society. The issues were complicated. There was polarization of members, while an effort was made in communications to sound normal. Letters poured in to the office from around the country. One member wrote: "All official communications from the present CMS office seem to imply that the splitting off of MAP from CMS was a natural and progressive step in the organization. The words are soft; the statements are logical; much of what is not said make this move appear to be a beneficial phase in the ministry of CMS." Many grassroots members wondered what was going on.

Dr. Markham Berry had been elected president of CMS after Gieser's resignation, and he tried—with the help of president-elect Paul Jorden—to calm the waters and express hope for the future. Dr. Gieser wrote to the members, "The events of the past few months bringing about two separate organizations have been a traumatic experience for all concerned. However, we trust this is God's plan. Now it behooves us all to use our influence, whatever it may be, to strengthen the vital ministries of CMS and MAP throughout the world."

Dr. Paul Jorden, who became CMS president in 1966, wrote: "I spent more time on my knees in prayer than I have at any other time in my life. Only by the grace of God did the Society survive. I felt at the time that the division of MAP from CMS was God's will for both societies. I believe the subsequent years have proved this to be true, since both societies have survived and flourished. However, in all honesty, I was disappointed in the manner in which the division occurred. It seemed that personalities took precedence over principle and great misunderstanding occurred."

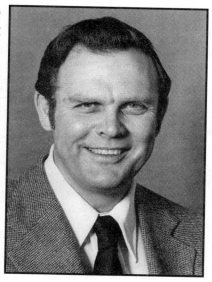

Dr. Paul Jorden,
CMS President, 1966-67

Today the two organizations are effectively serving God and have drawn closer to one another in mutual respect.

While MAP began functioning separately from CMS in November 1965, the official vote ratifying this separation was taken at the newly formed House of Delegates meeting in May 1967. The resolution was that "our relationship with MAP shall be the same as it is with any other organization of similar outlook and calling. We wish MAP well and desire to cooperate in all ways possible."

The House of Delegates had come into existence because for several years there had been building among CMS members the desire to have a voice in running the Society. A survey had indicated that eighty-four percent favored a democratically elected House of Delegates, perhaps fashioned after the American Medical Association. This would afford an opportunity for open discussion of issues, resolution of differences, affirmation of vision, and unity of purpose. Therefore, at the annual meeting of the CMS board of directors in 1966, a reconstruction process was initiated, with the prime responsibility to work out the change falling on newly appointed Executive Director, Dr. Walter O. Spitzer.

Dr. Spitzer, a physician from Canada already active in CMS affairs, was called to direct the Society in April 1966 while in a graduate program of hospital administration in Detroit, and acting as assistant

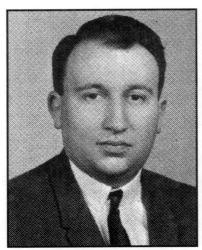

Dr. Walter Spitzer,
General Director, 1966-69

administrator for the Henry Ford Hospital. The son of missionary Bible translators in Paraguay, South America, Dr. Spitzer and his wife had also served as missionaries with the Grenfell Mission in Newfoundland and Labrador.

Dr. Spitzer moved to the Chicago area, focusing his administrative ability on the task of the Committee on Revision of Bylaws. The new system, effective January 1, 1967, was based on representation from sixteen electoral districts. In addition, delegates were to be selected from the missionary membership, students, and up to four members-at-large. Meeting once a year, the House would be the final policy-making body of the Society.

Prior to this, the president had been elected by the board of directors. But the new system called for the entire membership to elect, from candidates nominated by the House, a president who would serve a two-year term after two years as president-elect. A Board of Trustees would replace the Board of Directors The new board would be elected by delegates, and tasked with interpreting House policy and appointing a General Director.

Dr. Arthur Svedberg recalls, "I shall never forget helping to set up the auditorium the night before the first House. As I looked at it, I thought the Congress of the U.S. was going to meet there the next day, it was so impressive!"

The first assembly of the House of Delegates of the Christian Medical Society convened on May 5, 1967 in the Park Plaza Hotel, Toronto, Ontario, with president-elect Dr. Arthur H. Svederg calling the meeting to order. Trustees were elected, and the first man to take office as president-elect through balloting of the membership, Dr. William B. Kiesewetter, took office as Dr. Svederg moved on to become president.

CMS had kept as their responsibility what was to become known as "Medical Group Missions," which was originally called "Limited Group Missions." Earlier in the decade, society members in California had started a weekend ministry of flying medical missions to Mexico. Staff field man Mel Alexander described a typical trip: "We took off from Van Nuys and Long Beach airports and flew our airships, heavily loaded with equipment and supplies, to the nearest port of entry. Since a number of aircraft were involved, a rendezvous was necessary at the port of entry to discuss the locations, approach problems, etc., of the small airstrips and villages being served."

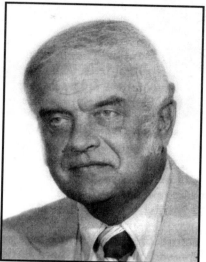

Dr. Arthur Svedberg,
first President with a
House of Delegates

Flying across arid desert to rough mountain areas of Mexico, clinics were set up in pole-and-mud huts, in school buildings, or under trees in small villages. It didn't take long for people to come. Each evening the village community gathered for the showing of public health films, entertaining films, and spiritual films like "The Life of Christ" or Moody Science films in Spanish.

The interest in such team efforts caught on, so Limited Group Missions officially became part of CMS ministries in 1967, after several years of projects in Mexico. The name was later changed to Medical Group Missions, known as MGMs through the years.

MGM's first major project occurred at Easter 1968, at the invitation of the government of the Dominican Republic. Dr. Gus Hemwall recalled: "I think we had at least 150 people who came on that first one. The President personally welcomed us at the airport where there was a large gathering of about 17,000 people. They had a caravan lined up to drive us to Puerto Plata. When we arrived there, we discovered our food had been highjacked! So for our stay we had to find beans and rice, which we could get locally."

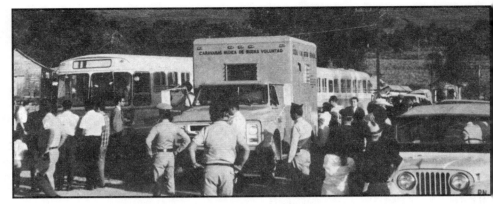

*The First MGM to the Dominican Republic is met
by an estimated 17,000*

According to Dr. Hemwall, the project experienced other problems, too. They ran out of water the first day as the unusually large group emptied the water tower. So someone was assigned to boil water all day on a two-burner stove, with rationing of a cup per person for each meal.

In spite of problems, the first Dominican project was well-received. An orthopedic surgeon was deeply moved when one woman who crawled around town on her hands and knees, reached up and thanked him for coming, realizing that nothing could be done for her, but so thankful that others could be helped.

But the local people were not the only ones reached. One of the pharmacists who had come along with a friend spoke up at the team's devotions: "You know I came here not quite realizing what this was all about. But having worked with the men in my group, I want to accept Christ as my Savior."

And thousands of people in the forty-nine villages visited heard the Gospel presented by team participants. Missionaries and national Christian workers from different missions cooperated, with follow-up of those who professed faith in Christ.

At the next House of Delegates meeting in San Antonio, MGMers gave their reports, focusing on some of the confusion of the first trip.

Yet their enthusiasm was obvious as they knew God would expand this ministry.

Then a visiting physician in the audience asked, "Say, would you come to Honduras?" Dr. Hemwall answered, "Well, all we need is an invitation from the government."

"I'll take care of that," the visitor replied. An ENT physician, he just happened to be the Vice President of Honduras!

In 1969, projects to Honduras and Haiti were added. Dr. Hemwall described the typical scene of the clinics: "We had thousands of people just swarming all over, no crowd control. It was just like everyone coming to a circus and trying to get in the door with free tickets! We seemed to sense that we were on the verge of something, but we also realized that the thing was just not well-managed."

Then help came. John W. Shannon, who had been living in the Dominican Republic for eleven years as a missionary, became the Director of MGM in 1969. As a result, MGM team members could look forward to taking their professional skills and sharing their faith in cross-cultural settings of need, even around the world, without the distraction of also having to handle the logistics of each trip.

Also during this decade CMS became more internationally involved with the founding of the International Congress of Christian Physicians (ICCP). By 1961, twelve countries had formed Christian Medical Fellowships, Associations, or Societies—Denmark having organized as early as 1897. Five of these groups led in planning for the formation of the ICCP, and for an international gathering. According to Dr. Paul Tournier, who represented France and Switzerland, this was a decision to "experiment" after a decade and a half of consideration on the part of leaders of the European fellowships. The purpose was for open exchange of views and for fellowship with Christian physicians from around the world.

The first ICCP Congress, held in July 1963 in Amsterdam, met its goal, bringing together some eighty participants from fifteen countries. The attendees enthusiastically agreed to hold a second

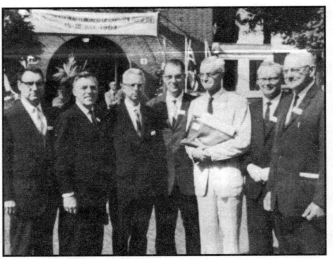

CMS members attending first ICCP:
(l. to r.) Drs. C. E. Koop, D. H. Nelson,
R. Blocksma, Executive Secretary J. R. Knighton,
Drs. V. Rambo, R. Jenson, and R. Ten Have

Congress in Oxford in 1966, with a request for a draft of a constitution and formal organization. A student group was also formed. At the Oxford Congress, with over 540 participants from thirty-four countries, the need for such an organization was confirmed. The representatives wanted to not only meet for international meetings, but also to assist doctors wanting to organize Christian fellowships in their own countries.

CMS-USA sent representatives to Oxford and was a charter member of the new organization, which became known in 1986 as the International Christian Medical & Dental Association (ICMDA) and the International Christian Medical & Dental Student Association (ICMDSA). International congresses continue to meet, now every four years, hosted by ICMDA groups worldwide.

Canadian physicians and dentists had played an active part in the American CMS almost from the beginning, with a number of chapters established in their provinces. But in 1969 the CMS of Canada was incorporated as an independent entity, in part to conform with Canadian tax laws regarding charitable organizations as CMS-Canada prepared to host the Third International Congress of Christian Physicians in Toronto in 1972. As a result, the membership of CMS-Canada grew. It has continued to be a strong organization, maintaining a cooperative relationship with CMS-USA.

CMS's increasing contact with missionaries brought a growing concern for their lack of access to good medical care because of rising costs. To address these needs, the Missionary Health Program of CMS was established in 1967, providing missionaries access to care at reasonable rates, with coverage anywhere in the world. This program went through various changes during it's approximately thirty years of existence, filling a crucial gap until other plans became available.

By the end of the 1960s, Christian leaders outside of CMS were beginning to look to the Society for help in facing the increasingly complex moral and ethical issues of the day. CMS was invited to co-sponsor, with *Christianity Today,* a symposium on "The Control of Human Reproduction." An interdisciplinary group of thirty scholars, representative of evangelical Protestantism, examined issues on the ethics of human reproduction from the perspectives of medicine, psychiatry, law, sociology, and theology. They met at the Wentworth-by-the-Sea Hotel in Portsmouth, New Hampshire on Labor Day weekend 1968. Lew Bird, Northeastern Field Director, took the CMS responsibility of helping organize this first symposium, as well as other symposia that would follow.

The interdenominational group included Christian leaders such as Dr. Harold J. Ockenga, Dr. Carl F. Henry, Kenneth Taylor, and Eric Fife. The delegates viewed the Bible as the final authority, hammering out a thousand-word declaration. Several months later Tyndale House published the Society's first major scholarly work entitled, *Birth Control and the Christian.* This included papers from the symposium, as well as other useful material.

In 1969, before leaving his post as CMS General Director, Dr. Walter Spitzer summarized his three-and-a-half years at the helm:

> When I accepted this position I was overwhelmed by the strong moral support with which the membership welcomed me. With that expressed encouragement as our principal asset, we began to rebuild CMS after the Society's rocky experiences of 1965. Regional directors have been hired, the Missionary Health Program was created, the Medical Group Missions ministry was fully developed, a scholarly Christian medical symposium was sponsored, and sister societies were encouraged and spawned in Latin America.

The 1960's can be described as a decade of tremendous expansion of the work, interrupted by division of ministries, followed by the adjustment to the resulting changes through refocusing of vision— all orchestrated by God through strong leaders intent on advancing the cause of Christ, worldwide, through the healing arts.

Chapter 5

Outreach And Growth:
The 1970s

The office of General Director was vacant for two years after Dr. Spitzer returned to Canada. As a result, it fell to Dr. Chris Reilly, then CMS president, to fill in at great personal cost of time and finances. He had a busy Ob/Gyn practice in New Jersey, but he ably extended himself to keep things in order, checking in at the Oak Park office and encouraging the regional directors on a regular basis. By 1970 CMS had recovered from the division of the mid-'60s; membership stood at 3,300, of which 800 were medical missionaries.

In 1971, Haddon Robinson, D.Th., Ph.D., was appointed General Director. Haddon's affiliation with CMS had begun in 1966 as a part-time Dallas Director. He had later become Southwestern CMS Regional Director while teaching practical theology at Dallas Theological Seminary. As General Director, he still continued as professor at the seminary,

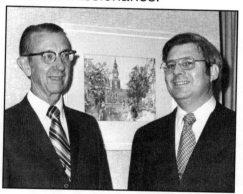

Drs. Gus Hemwall (l.) and Chris Reilly in 1971.

which meant periodic trips from Dallas to the central office in Oak Park, Illinois. Most weekends found Haddon, a gifted speaker, traveling as a public spokesperson for CMS. Members noted his disciplined habits as he was also able to fulfill multiple roles while also skillfully writing for the Society and editing the *Journal.* He and his wife, Bonnie, related well with participants in the family conferences. There was a rising tide of enthusiasm in the Society.

The day-to-day field work fell to the regional staff, and, as a CMS member said, "all without headlines." During this decade there were never more than six regional representatives at any one time. Theologically trained, they also kept abreast of what was happening in medicine. They were writing Bible study material and other litera-

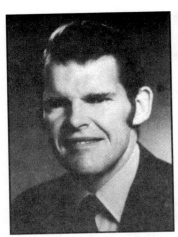

Dr. Haddon Robinson appointed General Director in 1971.

ture as publications were expanded. They devoted time to paperwork, correspondence, and organizing of meetings, including a growing number of conferences. There were many speaking engagements. They visited the medical students, started new groups, called on prospective members, and visited members in rural areas. As a result, their wives shared in the work as they were left behind to care for homes and children.

Sid Macaulay recalled what it was like to begin with CMS. "After a three weeks orientation in Oak Park and my appointment to the Southeast region, I planned an itinerary throughout the whole southeast in ten states. I planned to meet with all the members there. So from about the 20th of January to the 15th of June, I was on the road constantly. I didn't have time to look for a house, or to move our furniture, so my wife, Ann, did all those things."

Graduate work was growing, and chapters where added, especially in the cities. Chicago was an example of one very active chapter with many dinner meetings and special speakers.

While fellowship and service were high priorities for many CMS members, the regional staff saw the need for members to be more involved in outreach. They worked with the Board of Trustees to formulate a "CMS Statement on Evangelism," which was approved by the 1972 House of Delegates. The spring 1973 *Journal* was devoted entirely to the theme of evangelism, which was further emphasized in a series of pamphlets printed and made available for use in doctors' waiting rooms.

During the same year, the Society received a generous gift offer from the Tyndale Foundation to make copies of the *Living Bible*, a national bestseller at that time, available to physicians throughout the United States. A pilot program—nine CMS members in six states—distributed about 1,200 copies by simply offering them to friends and colleagues. More Bibles were distributed at medical conventions, and the decision was made to go ahead with this project. Tyndale provided an additional 15,000 copies. Student chapters also became involved in this outreach effort, with one group alone receiving requests for Bibles from at least 300 students. The follow-up was encouraging, with letters indicating that the Bibles were being read and studied.

Another outreach program of CMS that expanded rapidly in this decade was MGM. The principle that MGMs should pay for themselves was central to the success of this endeavor. Team participants covered their day-to-day expenses as well as all travel costs. Boxes of donated medicines and supplies were also brought along. Requests increased for specialty teams, such as surgery, dentistry, and ophthalmology, while the general medicine group projects continued to be filled. Through the years hundreds of thousands of patients have been treated by thousands of team participants.

The book *Million Dollar Vacations* by Madonna Yates (published by CMS in 1984), tells the story of the MGM ministry from its inception into the early '80s. The opportunity to take the family along on a "working vacation" was a strong drawing card. Family members didn't need professional medical experience in order to be general helpers, and for some teenagers, it was the first time they could see their doctor- parent at work.

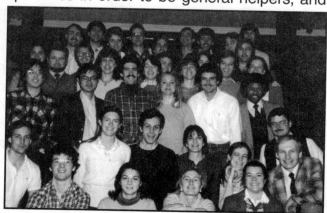

Sid Macaulay, fourth row, left, with a group of medical students

Dr. Curtis Drevets recalls that he went on the first MGM in 1968, took his wife, Jodie, on the second one, and then made sure that his three sons each went on two trips with them. He says, "These MGMs were very influential in our sons' lives. It gave them a view of another culture. They got to experience medicine (two of them are physicians), and they watched me in action as a doctor. Today I believe they are more interested in missions around the world because of their involvement with MGMs."

Often friends or colleagues, including office or hospital personnel, were invited to participate. For some, an MGM trip was the beginning of their own faith in Christ, as they witnessed Christians in action where the going was not always easy.

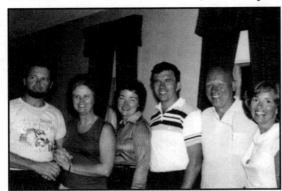

(l. to r.) Sid & Ann Macaulay, Pat & Ross Campbell and Lew & Carol Bird leading summer CMS camp

As the MGM work grew, the need for a headquarters became obvious. John Shannon found an unusual place to rent in 1970. It had been the summer palace of the former dictator of the Dominican Republic, President Rafael L. Trujillo, who had been assassinated in 1961. The problem was that the compound had been unoccupied for years, so it was in dilapidated shape. Also, it was isolated by miserable roads, situated on the rough seacoast some miles from the capital of Santo Domingo. Shannon found it with no electricity or water.

But John saw the potential. The Shannons used the last of their savings of $2,500 to start the repairs, and then scheduled two teams of young people to each come for two weeks in order to the prepare the facility to host its first medical clinic. The team members each paid $100, which was used to procure electrical wire and building materials.

Later the government gave permission to improve the facilities, and motel rooms were built around the swimming pool to accommodate teams. The fact that the pool was already there was a plus as the wild sea made the beach unsafe. Porches were enclosed to serve as dormitories and examining rooms, and the dining room and kitchen were readied.

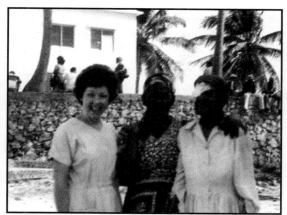

Patients wait with Madonna Yates in front of the MGM Headquarters, La Posada

John Shannon called this haven of healing on the sea "La Posada" (the inn), and for years it served MGM teams well, as the visiting personnel, as well as people seeking medical care, found refuge at the inn.

But there were frustrations when surgery had to be performed in remote places. In 1971 MGM received a grant, designated for a mobile surgical unit, from a foundation. Gifts came from others for the equipment. Haddon Robinson and John Shannon received the unit at the Presbyterian Hospital in Dallas. The hospital was responsible for the design of the surgical unit, with plans similar to a modern hospital operating room.

Over time, the MGM vision expanded beyond the Dominican Republic, Honduras, and Haiti. The first venture to Africa was to Liberia, West Africa. Dr. Gus Hemwall, immediate past president, and John Shannon visited Dr. Bob Schindler at the ELWA Hospital near Monrovia to lay the groundwork in 1973. As they sat around the dining table one evening, Gus shared his vision of bringing over 150 participants for the first visit. It was with some caution that the Schindlers reminded him that there were not many roads into the interior, nor many medical facilities in which to place team members.

However, plans moved ahead with determination. The Liberian government was most cooperative,

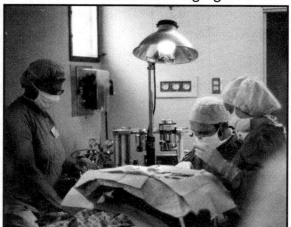

Donald Yates, assisted by Helen Shannon, operates in the Posada Surgery Trailer

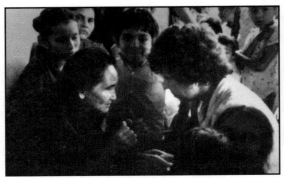

Woman expresses needs to Madonna Yates, R.N., on MGM trip

with the invitation extended by President William S. Tolbert. Dr. Nehemiah Cooper, a Liberian surgeon and the President's physician, arranged for teams to go into the government facilities, and Dr. Schindler took care of the mission contacts throughout the country.

In the final hours before the chartered plane was to come in January 1974, word was received in Liberia that they could not take off from New York because the oil embargo was forcing Liberia to refuse extra flights into their international airport for refueling. A hurried visit to President Tolbert's office opened the door at the last minute, and the flight was released.

The next day a TWA chartered plane landed at Robertsfield International Airport in Liberia with 164 MGM participants and friends on board. All usual customs regulations were waived. The visitors dropped their passports into a bag as they stepped from the plane, their luggage was piled onto the mission trucks, and they made their way to a caravan of vehicles that had been assembled to transport them to Monrovia, where the President of Liberia welcomed them, and they got their assignments before spreading out the next day.

The logistics of dispersing the group throughout Liberia were challenging. Mission and government planes had to carry people to remote spots, with costs graciously undertaken by the hosts. But everything was accomplished without major hitches, and the first MGM to Liberia was a success received by a very grateful people.

After the trip, many stories were recounted, but one incident in particular served as a vivid reminder, and an affirmation, of what CMS and MGM were all about. Five of the doctors were assigned to the ELWA Hospital. One doctor examined a man who complained of a headache, for which he was prescribed malaria treatment. But the man just sat there. Next, the visiting doctor gave him some aspirin. Still the man continued to just sit there. Finally, thinking that he must have missed something, the doctor asked, "Is there anything else?"

The man looked at him and asked, "Aren't you Christian Medical Society?"

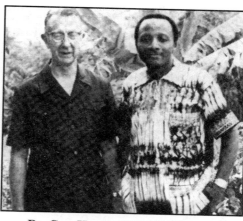

Dr. Gus Hemwall, MGM leader, with Mr. Bright, Minister of Health in Liberia

"Oh, yes," the doctor replied, and with pride he pointed to his name tag with "Christian Medical Society" printed on it.

"Aren't you going to tell me about Jesus Christ?" the man asked him. Gladly, of course, the physician described that the real reason he had come to West Africa was to bear witness to the love of Christ, for the patient as well as the doctor. But Bob Schindler recalls, "As the doctor shared with us, that struck us like a ton of bricks as we realized that we could have missed an opportunity as we were so intent on medical treatment – 'Aren't you going to tell us about Jesus Christ?'"

The first MGM to Liberia also helped launch another important min-

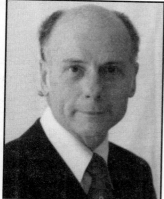

In Liberia Dr. David Stewart caught the vision of CMEs for missionaries

istry. Midway into the three-week MGM trip, CMS and MAP (which already had a respected ministry in supplying mission hospitals in Liberia), with Director Ray and Beth Knighton there, hosted a medical conference for missionary and national doctors from all over West Africa. Such internationally noted speakers as Dr. Dennis Burkitt and Dr. David P. Morley participated. This conference planted the seed in the mind of MGM participant and former missionary to Burundi, Dr. David Stewart, for what became the Continuing Medical Education Seminars (CMEs) for missionaries. He had returned to the States because of health reasons, taking a psychiatry residency, and continuing to help with mission needs through his practice in Kentucky. Dr. Stewart understood, more than many, the need for medical missionaries to keep up professionally with CME requirements, as well as to have a time for relaxation, and physical and spiritual renewal. It became his vision to see this happen.

As a result of Dr. Stewart's initiative, and with the enthusiastic support of other CMS leaders, the first CMS-CME program was held in 1978 during the third MGM to Liberia. Dr. Marvin Jewell, CMS president (1976-1978) and Dr. David Van Reken, pediatrician, then teaching at the Liberian Medical School in Monrovia, were recruited. Gerald Swim, Assistant Dean and Director of CME for the Louisville School of Medicine, helped with the accreditation of courses.

At the outset of this inaugural program, everything was going well. John Shannon was responsible for the MGM ministry at the same time as he was overseeing the CME symposium in Monrovia. But suddenly John, himself, was hit with a sudden and strange illness. Drs. David Van Reken and Marvin Jewell recall:

> *John was put in the ELWA Hospital just outside Monrovia. We had forty doctors hanging around, each teaching their specialty at the CME. There were many ideas on what to do, what tests to run, what antibiotics to give, etc. But when we realized there was no coordination of treatment, we appointed our Infectious Disease CME faculty member, Dr. Don Anderson from Michigan State University, to take charge. Progressive dehydration eventually led to the placement of a large-bore IV cannula in John's left arm and the administration of 16 liters of balanced solutions over about 24 hours, but John still went into renal shutdown. While drifting in and out of delirium, he recited to Gus Hemwall all the logistical and fiscal necessities related to finishing the MGM trip.*

> *It was decided that this disease wasn't something that John should fight in Liberia. God found three seats on an overbooked Air France flight to New York, and Don Andersen and Marvin Jewell accompanied him. However, a snowstorm in New York prevented the flight from continuing so an overnight stop was made in Dakar, Senegal to await clearance from New York. Marv and Don thought they might lose John as they cared for him in the terminal. However, the Lord opened up NYC, and the Air France flight was the first allowed to land. Shortly after that the snow started again,*

and the airport was closed. Dr. John Frame had been warned about the situation and had his residents waiting, whisking the three through customs and on to Columbia University Hospital. It was never determined just what John suffered from. Although weak and ill for many months, he made a complete recovery. Praise the Lord!

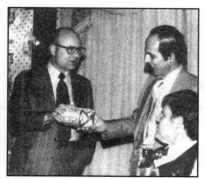

Dr. Marvin Jewell recognizes John Shannon at 1978 House of Delegates

When Dr. Jewell talked to General Director Robinson, Haddon shared that God had awakened him during the night, telling him to pray for John Shannon at the time of John's critical state. Haddon had been unaware of the situation, but realized that there must have been an acute problem with the MGM in Liberia, and so he prayed. Partly as a result of this health crisis and also because the MGM ministry was expanding so rapidly, John Shannon contacted Willie Hunter. Willie and his wife, Jan, were already enthusiastic missionaries in the Dominican Republic, and their gifts matched MGM's needs. They joined the staff to work with the Shannons.

The response from the missionaries attending the first CME conference was that this must continue. But the suggestion was made that Nairobi, Kenya would be a more accessible place for most participants. So in 1980, the Second International CMS-CME Symposium was held at Brackenhurst Baptist Conference Center, an hour out of Nairobi in the cool elevation of the Ngong hills, where the conference has met biennially since then.

Since CMS members were finding such a variety of special service opportunities, in 1973 the first commissions were set up to oversee these, with the task of bringing annual reports to the House of Delegates

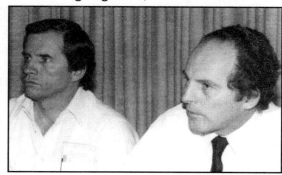

MGM Leaders Willie Hunter and John Shannon.

as well as periodic updates to the Board of Trustees. Three commissions were formed in this decade. Medical Group Missions, already very active, was named a commission in 1973, and was instructed to prepare short- and long-range goals for approval by the Trustees. The Medical Ethics Commission was also formed in that 1973 House meeting. After the pilot project in Liberia, the dream of David Stewart became an official CMS Commission on Medical Education for medical missionaries at the House of Delegates in May 1979.

The Medical Ethics Commission would provide a context for consideration of current issues in medicine and dentistry, addres-sing those issues from a Christian perspective. This commission would

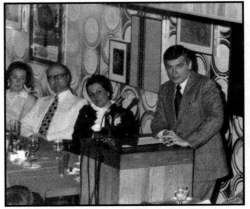

Senator Mark Hatfield addresses House of Delegates dinner –1975

serve the membership as a resource for literature, bibliography, and personnel. They would draft position papers to be ratified by the Trustees and House. There would be conferences and symposia. This commission would be a "think tank" to study and share information. Appointed to that first commission were Drs. David Allen, John Brobeck, Alastair Connel, Rob MacGregor, Robert Scheidt, Martin Singewald, and Robert Hermann, Ph.D., all of whom saw the tremendous need for CMS to help its members and others sort through the growing number of ethical issues. In the beginning, Lew Bird served as a coordinator for this commission. Through the years, the Medical Ethics Commission has continued to fulfill an important role in the Society, raising awareness of the need for the Christian perspective in ethics.

Notre Dame University was the site of a CMS-sponsored Symposium on Demonology in January 1975. The conference was called because of the increasing interest in occult activities in the United States. Participants represented the fields of psychiatry, biblical studies, missions, and pastoral concern. The response from participants was overwhelmingly positive. The papers submitted were published by Bethany Press in a book entitled *Demon Possession.*

CMS was invited to participate in a week-long symposium on the "Control of Man Through Human Engineering", held at Wheaton College in 1975, and sponsored by nine evangelical associations. They met to probe the ethical implications of this recent direction in medicine. This conference brought together distinguished scientists, theologians, psychiatrists, philosophers, and lawyers who prepared a landmark statement that, while reflecting a generally positive attitude toward research, issued a warning against the potential abuses of its application, and urged expanded "efforts to integrate Christian ethics with scientific concerns."

Then in 1979 CMS co-sponsored with Oral Roberts University School of Medicine an International Symposium on Whole Person Medicine at the University's campus. The holistic health movement was emerging in the U.S., with the blend of eastern religion with modern medicine. The Medical Ethics Commission worked hard on this project to help clarify the meaning of holistic health, emphasizing that true wholeness comes through a relationship with God through faith in Christ.

In the early 1970s, CMS wanted to begin the tradition of annually honoring one of their members with the "Servant of Christ Award." But as the Trustees looked for a person to honor that first year, they commented, "Frankly, the problem of selection is a difficult one. It is not that there are too few candidates, but too many. What standards should be used to single out one particular person for special recognition?"

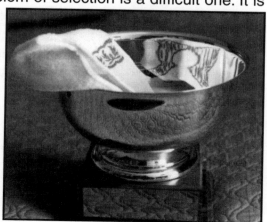

It was decided that the Servant of Christ award would honor a member whose servant-leadership lifestyle had demonstrated to both colleagues and patients the clear priorities of Christian disciple-

The Servant of Christ Award – Symbol of Servanthood

ship. The place of service would not be the most important factor. What was important was the professional and spiritual integrity of the service, the personal quality of truly caring for others, and the sense of ultimate loyalty rendered to Jesus Christ. The towel and basin award, a symbol of Christian humility and service, was first presented to Dr. Ernest Gregory at the annual House of Delegates meeting in 1972. Of Dr. Gregory, Haddon Robinson wrote in the *Journal*:

> *Whatever picture comes to your mind when you think of a surgeon, Ernest Gregory doesn't fit it. With hands like ham hocks and with features as rough as West Texas, he looks more at home on a construction crew than in an operating room. To many men and women on San Antonio's overcrowded West Side, however, Gregory is the greatest doctor they know. For hundreds of the poor in Mexico, he is the only doctor they know.... To those who work with him and to those who have been touched by his life, Dr. Ernest Gregory stands tall because of the love of Christ, he bows low to "wash the feet" of those in need.*

(Note: Lists of all award recipients are located in the appendix.

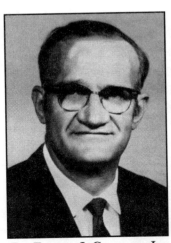

Dr. Ernest J. Gregory, Jr., first recipient of the Servant of Christ Award (1972)

By 1976, CMS was outgrowing its Oak Park, Illinois, headquarters, which had also fallen into disrepair. A committee began to search for a new location. Several sites and multiple factors were considered, including central location, nationally, with access to a major airport and medical centers. Close proximity to a John Hancock office was important for MHP. In early 1979, the committee recommended that CMS build a building in a business park under development on Gateway Boulevard in Richardson, a suburb of Dallas, Texas. The Trustees agreed, and the final decision was made by the House of Delegates. The new motto for CMS—"Gateway to Growth"—celebrated a new headquarters for more efficient operation and expansion of the growing ministries.

Dr. Len Ritzmann, chairman of the relocation committee recalls, "We got an architect who had built airports. He was now retired, but he was willing to oversee the construction of our building—the

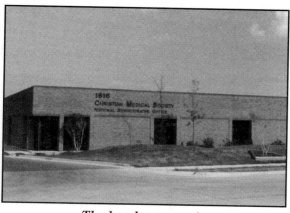

The headquarters in Richardson, Texas

resident foreman. The only thing we told him was that we didn't want the building to look like an airport! He got us good quality and saved us money, a token of love."

The cost of the building and move was to be approximately $500,000. Nearly $200,000 was on hand from the previous sale of the Oak Park property; therefore, fund-raising for the balance became a priority.

Haddon Robinson, General Director since 1971, had cautioned that he did not want the move to the Dallas area to be influenced by his residing there. In fact, as CMS was making its relocation decision, Dr. Robinson was making his decision to move to Denver to become the president of Denver Conservative Baptist Theological Seminary. So two important announcements were made at the May 1979 House of Delegates meeting—the relocation of the central office to the Dallas area and the General Director's resignation to be effective in September with his move to Denver. The announcement said, "While this came as a surprise, the Board saw this as an important opportunity for Haddon and for God's work in the world. If God is removing Haddon from CMS, He has a new man in mind for our General Director."

The Board invited Joseph Bayly, gifted writer and then vice president of David C. Cook Publishing Company, who had known CMS for some time—speaking at Society meetings and helping start student groups in several medical schools on the East Coast—to consider the position. Joe assumed his new role with CMS on August 1, 1979, with the understanding that he would continue with the publishing company and work for CMS half-time. So, as CMS was moving its offices from Chicago to Dallas, the Lord provided a part-time General Director whose office was in Chicago!

Bayly thought it a good idea to have a full-time Executive Director to take on the day-to-day responsibilities of running the Central Office in Texas. The name of Don Westra, J.D., was suggested, and Joe was enthusiastic on hearing this. The 1979 Thanksgiving letter to members announced that Westra had accepted the full-time position of Executive Director of CMS. He presently was Assistant Vice President for Medical Affairs at Ohio State University, where he had been active in a ten-year expansion program for the College of Medicine. With twenty-three years of military service, and as Executive Officer to the Surgeon General of the Air Force, the "Colonel" had supervised medical installations worldwide. While working at the Pentagon in Washington, D.C., he had earned a degree in business administration and law. A bonus was that the Texas State Bar had already licensed him. Don and his wife Mae (who had been a classmate of Bayly's at Wheaton) were to move to Dallas in March 1980.

In the meantime, the new building was completed in October 1979 and key staff moved down from Oak Park, while new employees were hired. It was difficult to leave behind faithful staff who could not make the move to Texas. The Chicago area had been the home of CMS for many years and the hub of much chapter activity. It was hard for some members to see the move occur.

Then, the midst of all of the activity in late 1979, word came of the disastrous Hurricane David, which pounded the Dominican Republic August 31 to September 1, followed by Hurricane Frederick three days later. The MGM headquarters at La Posada was not spared. The Shannon and Hunter families, with their staff, huddled under stairs in the women's bathroom as the waves relentlessly pounded the property, and the winds reached 180 miles per hour. Every window in La Posada was gone except one—the one in front of the bathroom door where the staff had been hiding.

Dr. John Paul, chairman of the MGM Commission and frequent team leader, immediately let MGM friends and the entire CMS membership know of the need for financial help as medicines, food, and supplies were being airlifted to the stricken country. The

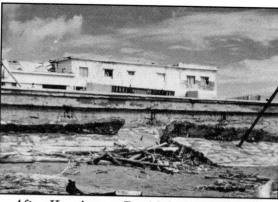

After Hurricanes David & Frederick, the surgery trailer was washed away. The Posada building is still standing.

response was generous, and MGM was able to help in a new way to bring relief to the poor.

According to the book *Million Dollar Vacations,* when Dr. Paul visited the area just eight days after the hurricanes, he admitted: "It will be impossible to restore our former base of operations. God has seen fit to take the greater part of this back to the sea.... We have lost our Posada."

Chapter 6

Changing Times for CMS:
The 1980s

$\mathscr{A}$s CMS settled into the new efficient one-story building in Richardson, Texas, an Open House and Dedication was held in conjunction with the Trustees meeting in January 1980. Joe Bayly, the General Director for just six months, had been kept busy learning the ropes of the new job as well as making decisions for the move. He had to hire new personnel in Texas to replace those who were not able to move from Oak Park. And the Trustees praised him for a job well done.

There had been other challenges to consider, too. Medical Group Missions Commission dealt with the loss of their headquarters in the Dominican Republic through the hurricanes in '79. The decision was made not to rebuild Posada headquarters, but to establish a warehouse in Santo Domingo for the time being.

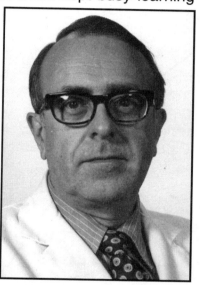

Dr. Leonard Ritzmann,
President (1979-81)

Membership giving had been gracious for those needs. The debt on the new building was wiped out by September 1980. Funds had poured in to help recover MGM's losses from the hurricane disaster as well as bring relief to the Dominican Republic. But there was a growing concern for significant operating deficits in other areas for CMS.

Then came the 50th Year Jubilee Celebration in 1981. Occasionally CMS USA and Canada joined for their annual meetings, and in May of that year, this was the case for the House of Delegates meeting. It was a beautiful setting with the background of snow on the moun-

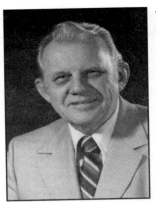

Don Westra, J.D., Executive Director, helped steer the course for CMS.

tains in Banff, Alberta, Canada. The scenery was spectacular. There was time for families to relax and play, and the conference in conjunction with the meeting focused on the lifestyle of the doctor, "Professional Priorities – A Christian Perspective." Dr. Kenneth Gieser, founder of CMS, was honored this Jubilee Year with the Servant of Christ Award.

But there were very important challenges at that meeting. Joe Bayly had served as General Director just less of two years. He had suffered a mild heart attack in April 1980 while on his way to a Regional ICCP meeting in Monterrey, Mexico. His traveling was curtailed over the next months, but he felt more pressure to carry on the duties while taking care of his health needs. His resignation was announced at that 1981 House of Delegates meeting. In the interim, he would continue to edit the CMS *Journal*. When he left, Bayly's faithful and effective leadership to the Society was acknowledged.

Dr. Art Svedberg, a Past President (1967-69), was appointed Acting General Director, to work closely with Executive Director Don Westra. Art had moved from his active practice in Ohio to be Medical Director of Shell Point Village retirement center in Florida. According to then President Dr. Jim Petersen, "Art accepted the call to work part-time, and without pay, until a new person could be found. He was a delight to work with, and was especially effective as liaison with the field staff."

It was fortunate that Joe Bayly had insisted on having an Executive Director to work with him, running the day-by-day affairs of the Society. Don Westra had come in March 1980, and already his administrative gifts were making a difference for the organization.

The financial picture presented at the House meeting was discouraging. Large deficits had accumulated over the prior two years. There were unexpected expenses with the move—getting the building ready, termination pay for those who stayed in Oak Park, addi-

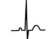

tion of new employees, and a change of General Directors at the end of '79. Dues collection was not up to date. Action had to be taken at the House in order to balance budgets in the future. One hard decision was to eliminate the position of the most recently hired field staff member, the Midwest Regional Director, Jim Barlow. His region was greatly disappointed, as they had not realized the seriousness of the situation. Fortunately, CMS was able to reinstate Jim to that position in May 1982, when the financial condition had improved.

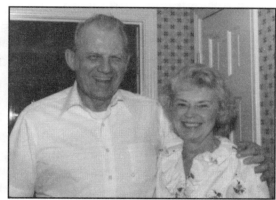

Don and Mae Westra opened their home to the CMS staff.

Jim Petersen says, "I recall those years as primarily ones of rear-guard action, retrenchment and struggling to move ahead. At the joint meeting with the Canadian CMS in snowy Banff in 1981, we were shocked by reports of a current deficit of $210,000, and news of the resignation of the General Director Joe Bayly. This was a devastating beginning for me as President, and I spent most of the night before my installation in prayer seeking wisdom and direction from the Lord, wondering if He had brought me to this place to oversee the demise of the Society. The heartsickness of those hours reminded me of the same feeling I had after my first night in combat in the war.

"But enter Don Westra. What followed was God at work through Don. CMS will never be able to know or appreciate all that he planned, organized, implemented and communicated to effect a recovery. These were very difficult times for him as he reduced staff and functions to fit income. But the miracle of it was that by the end of 1981, there was a surplus, completely erasing the whole general fund deficit of the two preceding years!"

Part of the recovery was the Planned Giving Program, which was devised and implemented by Don Westra. There also was a special Jubilee Year Fund Drive. But according to Don in his 1982 report to the House of Delegates, "The bottom line is that God answered prayers and rewarded efforts of many."

Don's wife, Mae, had the special gift of hospitality, and each month they invited the office staff to their home. This helped to solidify the team after the move and especially without a resident General Director at the time.

But the Westras also realized they were called to CMS when hard decisions had to be made and carried out for the Society. There were times of tumult. And Don recalls how his helpmate also had the gift of encouragement, leaving notes for him. One he shared:

> *To my strong rock upon whom I lean –*
> *"It is not for us as passengers of a ship to meddle with*
> *the chart*
> *and compass. Leave that all-skilled Pilot alone with His*
> *own work.*
> *He will safely steer the ship through the storm and lead*
> *us safely into the harbor."*
> *Even the rock has to have a greater rock to hold it up!*
> *Yours always, Mae*

But then the CMS family was shocked and saddened with the news that Don and Mae's youngest son, Jim, just 21 years old, died October 26, 1981 following a tragic car accident. He had already become a "friend of the Society," by volunteering as a computer operator in between his work schedule.

Don said, "Amid the tears and the wonderful glory of God's grace, Mae and I covenanted to establish the 'James S. Westra Memorial Fund.'" This was the first endowment fund established for CMS. The income from the fund was to be used to "foster, encourage and promote Christian fellowship among students in the medical and dental professions and to aid the ministry of Christian medical missionary activities." Through the years, numerous scholarships have been awarded to medical/dental students to go to serve short-term in mission hospitals, and they have told their stories of the lasting influence to serve Christ.

By January 1982 the Board of Trustees appointed the next General Director, Dr. L. Arden Almquist. He came as the first full-time General Director in twelve years. President Petersen said, "Arden Almquist, M.D., comes to us as one of our own members, with proven

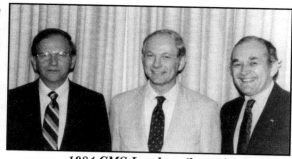

1984 CMS Leaders (l. to r.):
Dr. James Peterson, Past President;
Dr. Curtis Drevets, President;
Dr. Robert Schindler, President-elect

leadership skills and service achievements, to provide leadership to CMS in a time of unprecedented challenge. He is a practical man of God."

Arden had trained in theology and medicine and had had a career in missions and administration. He had served as a medical missionary in the Congo from 1952 to 1962, and following that had served in administration in the church's mission work. At the time of appointment he was Director of Medical Education at Baptist Memorial Hospital in Kansas City, Missouri, while pastoring a church there.

The 1980s saw frequent changes in leadership. After only a year, CMS announced with regret that, for health reasons, Dr. Arden Almquist would step aside as General Director in 1983. Dr. Curt

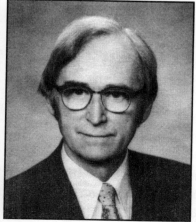

Drevets, who had become President, reported that Arden was asked then to take the new position of Director of Missions. Curt Drevets said, "This is a position of his first love. Arden showed us a tremendous need to expand CMS services to our missionary colleagues." In the meantime, Don Westra, after three years as Executive Director, was asked to take responsibilities as General Director for the next year, while a search was made for the new Director. Art Svedberg would direct the expanded field staff.

Dr. Arden Almquist, General Director (1982-1983)

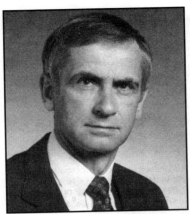

Edwin Blum, Th.D., General Director (1984-87)

When a Director would be found, Dr. Westra could move on to direct and develop the Planned Giving Program for a number of years in a part-time position.

By February 1984, the Trustees appointed a new General Director, Edwin Blum, Th.D., who took office in April. Dr. Blum was then professor of New Testament at Dallas Seminary, so a move to the area was not necessary for him. He had known about CMS as he was a friend of Haddon Robinson, a past General Director. He also had pastored churches, and at the present time was a teaching elder at Trinity Fellowship in Richardson, a church that he and CMS member Alan Hull had started. He also was leading a large Bible study for business and professional people in Dallas.

Dr. Drevets introduced him with these words, "Dr. Blum is an outstanding leader. He not only brings to CMS a solid record of academic and theological achievement, but he also shares our vision of being a healing witness in a hurting world." Blum had a rapid grasp of CMS history and a steady hand to help stabilize areas of need. Under his leadership, end-of-year financial reports carried a positive balance. But it came as a surprise three years later, after the May House of Delegates meeting in 1987, that Dr. Blum sent a letter of resignation to say that he was leaving Dallas to move to California to assume an administrative position there.

So again it was time to look for another General Director, and in the meantime, the new President, Dr. Mayo Gilson, in Ob/Gyn practice, only four weeks into his presidency, often had to commute from Oklahoma City to take care of CMS business. He was an encouragement to the field staff and sought to strengthen a spirit of love and fellowship in the Society. But again, near the end of Mayo's term as President, the CMS family was saddened with the word of a personal tragedy for the family of another one in leadership. The Gilsons' oldest son Brent had been fatally injured in a car accident caused by a drunken driver. Mayo wrote, "I can't begin to adequately describe the ministry of the members of CMDS in person, by letter, by telegram, by phone calls and countless other avenues of love that they poured out upon us in our time of deepest grief and need." A "Brent W. Gilson Memorial Fund" was set up to honor the memory of Brent, who had been completing college and planning to enter seminary.

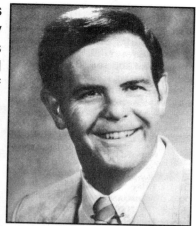

Dr. Mayo Gilson,
President (1987-89)

The "CMS Founders Fund" was set up in memory of Dr. P. Kenneth Gieser, who died in 1987. It was to be a revolving loan fund, interest free, for medical/dental students in need. The Gilson Memorial Fund was the first designated fund put under that fund. Others scholarships named during the decade were the "Anthony D. Vance Scholarship" and the "James Owen Scholarship" funds.

Hal Habecker, D. Min., was appointed as the next General Director in December 1987. He was no stranger to CMS. While in seminary, he had had a ministry to doctors through a class at First Baptist Church in Dallas. Then the church had asked him to come on to their staff to work with doctors when he finished training.

Hal recalled, "I went to visit Haddon Robinson because I had heard about CMS. 'Tell me what you know about working with doctors,' I said. We talked for two hours. And so that's when I started getting involved with the medical school and dental school, and we started all kinds of things all over Dallas. That was in 1978, after I finished seminary."

But Joe Bayly had also had a part in Hal's story. "Joe spoke at a Youth for Christ conference when I was in high school, and I had some time with him. When I was at Dallas Seminary, Joe came down for a weekend conference, and I asked if I could be Joe's host. When he left, he said, 'Let's keep in touch.'"

When Joe became General Director, Hal contacted him. And Joe said, "Hal, you've got to help us." So Hal came on, first as part time for Dallas work while still at the church, but then full-time, to be South Central Regional Director for six years and a Field Director under General Director Ed Blum for one year.

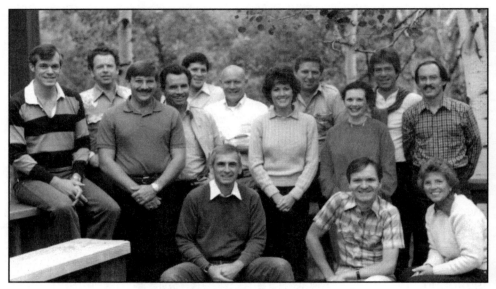

1984 Field Staff Meeting in Colorado.
(l. to r.) Seated: Ed Blum, Joe Ludders, Marti Ensign.
Standing: Doug Knighton, Sid Macaulay, Ron Lively, Willie Hunter,
Hal Habecker, Lew Bird, Brenda McFarlane, Chuck Hooker,
Sharon Smith, Jim Barlow, and Mike McLaughlin.

So coming with experience with CMS, a love for people and for ministry, and a vision for what God could do through Christian doctors, Hal Habecker was the man to effectively lead the organization on into the '90s. The position of General Director was to finally be filled for several years by one person.

During all these changes, what else was going on in the organization? Jim Petersen, as President, saw the need for a long-range plan to be developed to get things back on course. He named a Long-Range Planning Committee, which made a major contribution for the future years.

President Petersen, along with other leaders of national religious organizations, was privileged to receive an invitation to join

President Reagan for a meeting at the White House on April 13, 1980, to hear about the President's Task Force on Private Sector Initiatives. Petersen had the opportunity to share how the Christian Medical Society, then with 5,000 members, had found ways to do this. Information about CMS which was distributed said, "Our motto *'Non ministrari sed ministrare'* which means 'Not to be ministered unto but to minister' is taken from Mark 10:45. Following Christ's example, we seek to serve our fellowmen." The MGMs and CMEs for missionaries were given as examples.

Coming back from this meeting, Jim wrote in his report, "We know that many CMS members provide volunteer health services on an individual basis here in the States, but CMS has little in the way of nationally or regionally organized efforts." Perhaps this started more consideration about possibilities in domestic missions.

Hal Habecker, D.Min., General Director (1987-1993)

This was also a decade of tremendous change in the medical profession. As President Drevets noted in his report to the House in '85, "As I listen to and observe my colleagues, I sense much fear, insecurity, and uncertainty. There is fear over outside intrusion into our profession by big government, corporate medicine, insurance agencies, and hospital administrators. There is fear of the falling workload and income, [fear] over malpractice, and increasing distrust by patients. There is also the ever-increasing body of new scientific knowledge and the pressure of how to keep up with even a small corner of this." How could CMS help members with these challenges?

In addition, there still were the missionary members to be considered, far removed from the changing medical atmosphere in America. Dr. Almquist had moved on to another ministry, leaving a need in the office for help with missions.

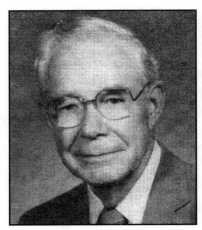

Dr. John S. Bagwell,
Missions Coordinator

Dr. John Bagwell, long-time CMS member who lived in Dallas, met this need in 1985 and became part-time Missions Coordinator. Retiring from a busy forty-four years of internal medicine and gastroenterology practice, Bagwell did not want to be idle. His first priority was to publish the monthly newsletter "Medicine SCAN" for medical missionaries, containing brief, pertinent abstracts from medical journals. This has continued through the years. His vision included sending appropriate specialists' journals and tapes. He wanted to send spiritual helps. And he looked for ways to help missionary children in the States, away from parents, looking for physicians and dentists willing to offer their services here. He set up a registry of practice and training opportunities for doctors returning to the States, as well as places of service abroad for stateside members. Jim Barlow, Th.M., Midwest Regional Director, set up Misson-Link, putting students in contact with missionary members.

Dr. Bagwell did much to expand this ministry for which he felt such concern, and upon his sudden death in October 1987, his son said, "He was a missionary at heart, though he never went overseas." He had not been idle.

Many helped to keep the focus on the priorities of the CMS ministry during changing times. There still were new directions to move forward in the 1980s and more stories to tell of God's leading.

Chapter 7

New Directions:
The 1980s Continued

There were challenges and changes, but there also were new directions for CMS to pursue with God's leading.

Probably one of the most notable expansions in the 1980s was the addition of new commissions, where members found more opportunities to use their gifts in service. Three commissions had been formed in the '70s and each was growing in its ministry.

The oldest, the MGM Commission, continued to take growing numbers of teams to Central and South America, and occasionally to Africa. John Shannon and Willie Hunter worked well together, so when John and Sheila Shannon returned to missionary work in the Dominican Republic after 14 years with MGM, Willie Hunter moved on to be the Director in '83.

But while MGM teams were going, there was something special happening again in the

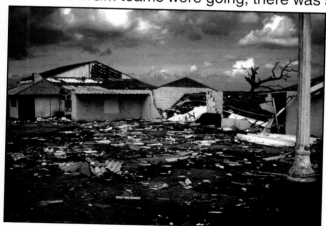

Damage caused by Hurricane David

Dominican Republic. In March '85 a new ambulatory care center, designed by MGM, was opened there, twenty-two kilometers outside Santo Domingo in densely populated Los Alcarrizos. The Dr. Elias Santana Center, named in memory of an outstanding Dominican Christian physician, was self-supporting apart from donated supplies, medicines, and the MGM volunteers. The remainder of the Hurricane David fund had helped to build this,

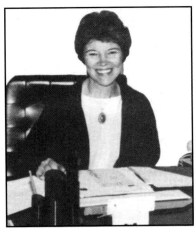

Janice Hunter,
Administrator of the
Dr. Elias Santa Center

and gifts also came from the Evangelical Medical Aid Society of Canada. Other designated gifts helped equip the center. The Center was owned and operated by Centro Cristiano de Servicios Medicos, a Dominican non-profit corporation with an eye clinic in Santo Domingo.

The design of the building was practical, as teams had learned much from seeing up to 1,000 patients a day in various settings. There was plan for ease of crowd movement, covered waiting areas, and outside rooms for eye exams and dental work. There were two operating rooms, which could be converted to four. There were two wards for post-op care, plus a pharmacy and laboratory. A lovely chapel was nearby, also used for staff meetings and education. Down the road, the former Child Evangelism camp was remodeled and called "Chicken Hilton," providing dorm facilities and rooms for couples for the MGM teams.

The poor received quality medical care. Jan Hunter, Willie's wife, ably served as Hospital Administrator. The core staff, including physicians, was Dominican; a 1989 report said the MGM volunteers worked along with the staff of eighty. Dr. Carlos Gomez, who had

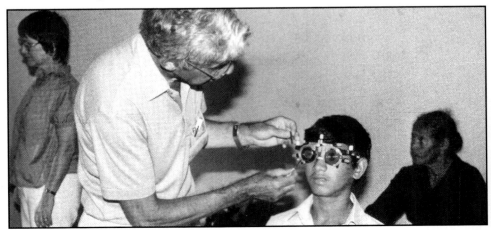

Ophthalmologist at work during a MGM

helped MGM projects for ten years, first as a translator-helper, and now as a physician, directed the program. Basic health teaching was taken to the surrounding villages.

To meet an apparent need, an ophthalmology residency program was started. Dr. Juan F. Batlle had returned to his Dominican home after a residency in the States where he had become a Christian, and he joined the staff as Instructor in Ophthalmology.

Florida Christian ophthalmologist, Dr. James P. Gills, had a dream that fit right into this. He believed that restoring vision was a wonderful way to help people in poor circumstances to regain their independence and become productive. He formed the Cataract Teaching Foundation to establish facilities to train eye doctors. When he learned of the MGM vision, he directed his efforts to help with the equipment needed, networking with others. The Santana Center was equipped with laser, ultrasound, operating microscopes, slit lamps, autoclave, and so forth for the training of residents as well as the care of the needy. This was a wonderful place for MGM ophthalmologists to come to teach as they treated patients waiting for vision to be restored.

The Continuing Education Commission continued to take faculty lecturers to Kenya every two years for the teaching conferences for medical missionaries, offering CME credits which were required for continued licensure in the States. But in order to meet similar needs of missionary doctors in other parts of the world, the Fourth International Symposium in Continuing Education sponsored by CMS and the University of Louisville School of Medicine was held in January 1983 at the Golden Sands Baptist Assembly grounds on the Straits of Malacca in Malaysia. This conference

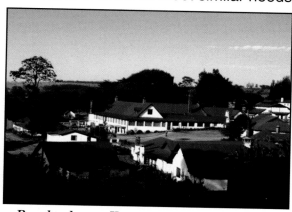

Brackenhurst, Kenya - a beautiful spot for missionaries to get their CME

continued to be held there on alternate years from Kenya's conference until 2001, when it was moved to Thailand.

Each year saw growing numbers of attendees to both places, moving up each year with "the largest ever," and ending the decade with "record attendance." Not only did the participants appreciate the excellent lectures by visiting faculty who paid their own way, but they highly valued the times to exchange ideas with one another in the "Serendipity" sessions— where they really got practical about how to do what was needed even if you didn't have everything you needed. The spiritual life speakers refreshed tired workers. The packed schedule was interspersed with tea times, meals, and late night chocolate where participants continued to share on a personal level. The spouses had a special program, and children were well taken care of with their activities planned.

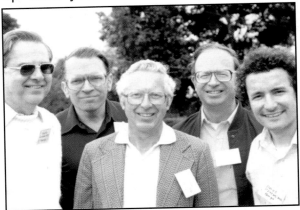

CMDE attendees from Tenwek Hospital (l. to r.) Drs. Graber, Wesche, Steury, Morris and Stevens.

Some who went said, "Sometimes we feel like a sponge out of water. Coming here to soak up all we can–the scientific knowledge and the spiritual inspiration...is just fantastic."

Another participant said, "After seven years on the field, giving out all the time, it is wonderful to come to a place like this and just take it all in."

Essential participants, too, were those not seen at the conference. They were the doctors who came from the States to cover for the mission doctors in remote hospitals so they could attend.

Four new commissions were started in the 1980s. When Dr. Leonard Ritzmann was President ('79-'81), he called for an Ad Hoc

Committee for Evangelism Within Health-care, as this was dear to his heart. A national conference on evangelism was held at the close of the 1982 House of Delegates meeting in Dallas. Dr. Paul Brand, recipient of the Servant of Christ award that year, opened the Conference. The "News and Reports" said, "Those who attended heard a deep personal testimony from a fellow Christian who is firmly convinced of the need for Christian men and women in medicine and dentistry to persuade others to follow Christ by the testimony of their *lifestyle* as used by the Spirit of God."

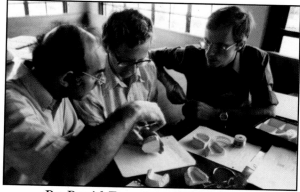

Dr. David Topazian, CMDE dental faculty, gives instruction.

The 1983 House of Delegates gave official Commission status to this thrust for evangelism. By 1984 a packet of materials was prepared to be available to members, and Dr. Ritzmann, Commission Chairman, asked the membership for vignettes of how they use tools for their own personal evangelism. A book, *Evangelism for Medical and Dental Professions,* was published, and the Commission continued to spur the membership to use opportunities for outreach to patients, colleagues and friends, sharing the love of Christ. In later years the Commission was discontinued, as their work was brought under the total ministry of the Society in view of the organization's affirmation that evangelism (and discipleship) should permeate *everything* the Christian doctor does.

More attention was also directed to healthcare for the poor in our nation. Dr. Robert Schindler was President when a Task Force on Healthcare for the Needy was formed in 1985, with Peter Boelens, M.D., as Chairman. According to Schindler's report after attending their first "think tank" session, "Goals were set aimed at building an informed membership concerning health needs of the economically depressed and what Christians are already doing to meet these needs." This became a committee in 1986.

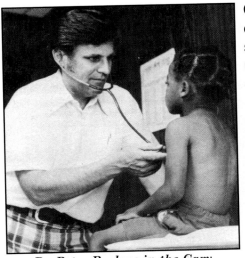

Dr. Peter Boelens in the Cary Christian Health Center

CMS wanted to offer support and encouragement to those already serving the poor, and a questionnaire to the membership indicated that many were already finding different, creative ways to serve, often working with their churches or other agencies. An example of one already very involved was the Chairman himself, Dr. Peter Boelens, who was then head of The Luke Society. In 1971 he, with his wife Eleanor, began a medical-evangelistic ministry to needy delta residents of Cary, Mississippi, an area of poverty. Sixteen years later, they were still working there. A pediatrician, Boelens noted the elevated infant mortality rate, which declined as a health program was initiated. There also was the addition of a family dental clinic and social and spiritual programs.

Other examples of work already being done appeared in the *Journal*, and a slide program was prepared depicting healthcare for the poor, featuring twelve CMDS members who did it their own distinct way. Art Jones, M.D., found his practice in the inner city of Chicago. He and his wife Linda had planned to go overseas after training, so in his fourth year of medical school they went to Liberia. He said, "Strangely enough, it was while we were there that we sensed a call to work in the inner city of Chicago. The missionaries said it would definitely be more difficult than working in Liberia."

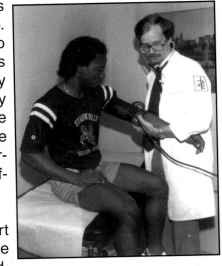

Dr. Art Jones saw the need for Chicago inner city health care.

The Jones's had been in on the start of the Lawndale Church located in the inner city, while Art had been a medical student at the University of Illinois

College of Medicine. So when they returned from Liberia, they decided to move into that neighborhood. The church became interested in starting a health clinic while he was in internal medicine residency. So Art looked for direction from other organizations such as the Christian Community Health Fellowship, knowing that medical school didn't train doctors for this. He met others working with the underserved, and learned from them. The result was the founding of the Lawndale Christian Health Center with Jones as Medical Director.

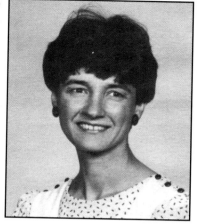

Dr. Carolyn Klaus founded Koinonia Health Services in Philadelphia

Over in Philadelphia, Dr. Carolyn Klaus found working in the heart of one of the most economically depressed regions was her calling. She had been a volunteer on an evangelistic project during the summer of 1982, and she was challenged to return to look at the health needs. Dr. Klaus founded Koinonia Health Services in 1985 to help to meet the physical as well as spiritual needs of that community. In 1987 this outreach became known as the Esperanza Health Center (translated "Hope"), reflecting the ethnic background of the area.

The Committee was officially named the Domestic Missions Commission in 1988. Moving from finding out what members were already doing, they continued to make CMS an advocate for healthcare for the poor and a facilitator of means through years ahead.

The Ethics Commission continued to sense the challenge of frequent new ethical issues faced by the profession, and they worked at helping the membership look carefully at these through a biblical perspective. Hal Habecker spelled this out in the booklet, *Opinions on Ethical/Social Issues,* "The principles include the sanctity of life, the importance of serving and honoring patients, and the necessity of gathering scientific information and weighing options objectively." A bimonthly *Bioethics Newsletter* was launched and sent out for several years. Articles appeared in the *Journal*, often written by David L. Schiedermayer,

M.D., who at the time was the Associate Director for the Center for the Study of Bioethics, Medical College of Wisconsin, in Milwaukee.

CMS helped to sponsor another ethical symposium, with the American Scientific Affiliation, held at Gordon College in June '88. The subject was the "Imago Dei: Relating Man in the Image of God to the Health Sciences – Theological, Scientific, and Clinical Implications," bringing together theological and bioethical considerations. Objectives included exploration of the debate over human personhood, examination of ethical principles and landmark legal precedents, discussing implications of modern technology in respect to the sanctity and dignity of the patient, and providing guidelines.

By the end of the decade, a number of statements had been formulated by the Commission, and debated and ratified by the House of Delegates. While these statements were not to be binding on the membership, they came from shared faith and a desire to serve Christ in the profession. Hal Habecker wrote, "The Christian physician and dentist grapples with problems which would baffle even Solomon. But One far greater than Solomon is with us. As always, unto the end of the age, He walks with us, helps us make the right decisions, and reaches out through us to heal the sick." The statements formulated by the end of the 1980s included opinions on:

- *Abortion*
- *Aids*
- *"Baby Doe"*
- *Euthanasia*
- *In Vitro Fertilization*
- *Reproductive Technology*
- *Use of Fetal Tissue for*
   Experimentation & Transplantation*

There was another urgent need. Christian doctors and their families were not immune from the noted societal changes in priorities for marriages and families, and some were in crisis. Because of the stress involved in their profession, there was a call for help designed especially for medical and dental families. Drs. Bob Schindler and Charles Crown, psychiatrist in Colorado, talked long about this need while at an ICMDA meeting in Cancun, Mexico in '86. An Ad Hoc Committee on Marriage and the Family was formed that same year to address these issues, and Dr. Crown was appointed chairman.

The initial group included six physicians whose practices showed special interest in marriage and family issues, and it was significant that they brought their spouses to the planning meeting. They chose three levels to consider: 1) Prevention of marriage problems and preparation for a Christian marriage; 2) need for enrichment; and 3) need of therapy.

Plans were made for two marriage growth conferences to be held in 1987, and additional conferences in 1988. There would also be a two-week marital therapy program for couples at Marble Retreat Center, run by CMS member Dr. Louis McBurney, in Colorado before the May 1988 House of Delegates meeting. And a list of therapists for referral would be prepared to encourage CMS field staff to use when members requested help. The need was being addressed, and the Marriage and Family Commission (named in 1988) continued to offer Marriage Growth Conferences and other valuable helps through years ahead.

Then another call came for help. It was following the '87 National Convention in New Orleans when Dr. Schindler had turned the President's gavel over to Dr. Mayo Gilson. As Schindler walked out of the hotel, Dr. Roberto Rodriguez, President of the CMS of Mexico

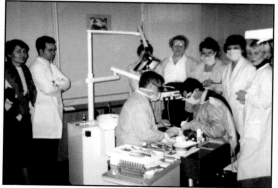

A COIMEA trip - Drs. Neal Smith (l.) and David Stryker (r.) teach dentists in Russia.

and friend of many, challenged him with a new thought. He said, "Your doctors have so much to share in professional knowledge and skill. There are so many around the world who could benefit from their teaching." His challenge was, "Why doesn't CMS-USA send your members to teach national physicians and dentists in their own countries?"

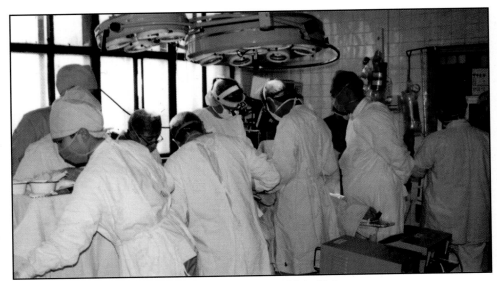
Early COIMEA Teaching Trip

Bob recalls, "We talked more about this, and concurred that it was a great idea and that we would both pray about this." Bob shared this with others. The Commission on Medical Education felt that they could not take on this added responsibility, as their plate was already full with their commitment to education for missionaries. The MGM Commission said it would not fit into their program. So in 1988 the Trustees formed an Ad Hoc Committee on International Medical Educational Affairs, which became known as COIMEA, with Schindler as chairman.

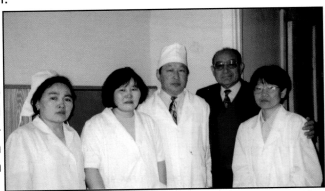

The goal was to provide medical and dental educational opportunities around the world for national physicians and dentists in their own countries through CMS-USA volunteers. The purpose was also to encour-

COIMEA Representative, Dr. George Mikhail with maternity staff in Mongolia

age Christian national doctors and to be a witness for Jesus Christ to non-Christian colleagues. There would be places where Christian Medical/Dental Fellowships could be encouraged or even some started. Volunteers would find that they would build relationships with mutual respect in learning from those in other countries.

The first contacts were made with the Christian Medical Fellowships of the International Christian Medical/Dental Association (name changed from the ICCP to ICMDA in 1986) in the countries that would most appreciate this help. The response to inquiries was very positive, and so the needs were made known to CMS members. Within a short time, the list of countries grew rapidly.

By 1989 individual doctors went on pilot projects. An invitation came from Poland's new Christian Medical Fellowship and Dr. Stephen Dunn, pediatric surgeon, was the guest lecturer who went to speak on "The Ethics of Transplantation." The door opened for teams to return to teach in medical centers in Poland through the following years, with opportunities to also share their faith as the CMF of Poland also arranged meetings inviting their colleagues.

George Miller, an Ob/Gyn specialist, traveled to Kathmandu, Nepal to teach at a maternity hospital. He was able to take a portable ultrasound unit along to enhance his teaching, which was particularly useful in this country which did not have the equipment at that time. Nepal has continued to host COIMEA trips.

Upon invitation, Dr. Richard Gieser went to the Vellore Christian Medical College and Hospital in India as a visiting lecturer in their Department of Ophthalmology. And a month later in '89, Dr. J. Leslie Walker provided the honored Ida Scudder Memorial Lecture. As an Ob/Gyn specialist, he lectured and demonstrated operative laparoscopy and hysteroscopy. It was concluded that the teaching projects in India were successful and COIMEA teams have continued going there.

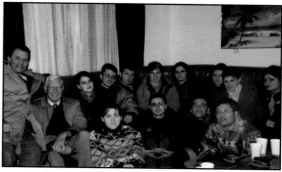

Albanian medical students during a COIMEA team's visit

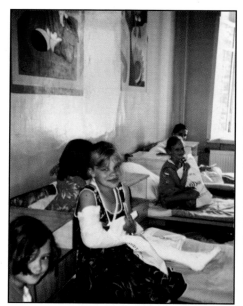

During a COIMEA trip to Russia, the gospel was presented and care packets were given.

Plans were already being laid for trips early in '90 to Romania, where Dr. Jon Askew would take a team and find a tremendous response from a fledgling Christian Medical Fellowship. So COIMEA was off and running, and became an official Commission in 1991. Opportunities opened up for individuals or teams to go. The settings were varied all around the world, from one-on-one teaching in rural areas to academic teaching in medical/dental schools and medical centers.

Through the years, COIMEA has expanded to give members who have an interest in teaching a place to go and teach, while also sharing their faith in Christ.

During this decade, CMS-USA had several opportunities to encourage the development of CMS Mexico. It was only natural for a relationship to develop as the national office was in Texas at the time. Hal Habecker recalled, "I remember meeting Dr. and Mrs. Rodriquez at the CMS office back in 1981. We got involved in sending speakers to their national meetings in '83, '84, and '85, and they were great times of fellowship and sharing. Students from several of the Mexican medical schools came to Texas for our leadership conferences, and our students traveled to the Mexico meetings as well. In fact, one medical student from Southwestern Medical School met his future wife at one of those meetings."

In the '80s doctors were again encouraged to form Specialty Sections to provide support to CMS members within their own specialty. Meetings could be educational as well as for fellowship. The Psychiatry Section had formed more than 20 years earlier, and was very active. Some years they held a full week of activities in conjunction with the annual meeting of the American Psychiatric

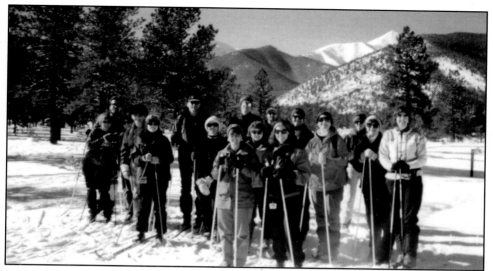
Singles ski trip at Deer Valley

Association. The Orthopedic Section was the next to be established in 1983; Dermatology in 1985.

Also In 1985, a new conference was instigated in the U.S. This was the Winter Singles conference, meeting the first year at Deer Valley Ranch in Colorado. They called it "an experiment," wondering if it might become a yearly event. And it was proven to be a good idea, with some even finding life partners through this!

An important international convention was held in 1986, the Eighth International Congress of Christian Physicians and Dentists, meeting in Cancun, Mexico in August. The hosts were the Christian Medical Societies of Mexico and the USA. The Mexican CMS committee was most gracious, and unique was the invitation from Mexico to host two hundred visiting doctors in different parts of the country for short periods of time before or after the Congress, with no charge to the guests.

East Germany was still under communist rule at that time, but their delegates wanted badly to come to Mexico. They were required to fly to Cuba on their way. At the conference, people prayed as these delegates had not arrived as the conference opened. A day later they received a wonderful warm welcome. Their clothes had been stolen en route, but attendees from other countries graciously took

care of that for them. And in the meeting, the East German delega-
tion gave a stirring testimony of God's grace through difficult times.

At this congress meeting, the name of the organization was
changed from International Congress of Christian Physicians
(ICCP) to the International Christian Medical & Dental Association
(ICMDA). And the student arm was named the International
Christian Medical & Dental Student Association (ICMDSA).

Also, the CMS national office in Texas served as a convenient platform
to encourage all of Latin America. Hal Habecker made several trips to
help in the development of national societies. Dr. Evert Bruckner played
a strong role in this as well. In 1988 Hal Habecker and MGM Director
Willie Hunter traveled to Paraguay and Argentina for one of their early
ICMDA regional meetings for southern South America.

Meanwhile, CMS also continued to encourage the development of
student and national ministries around the world. Hal took a small
number of students with him to Egypt in '85 for an international student conference. Some of the students who participated in those
trips are now serving Christ as missionaries around the world. In the
U.S., there was a strong national student ministry. This gave birth to
two national student conventions in 1988 and 1989 held in Dallas at
Dallas Baptist University, with 300-400 students attending each

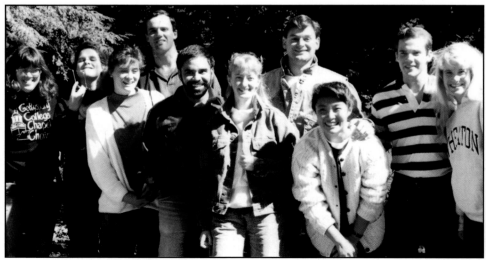

Students at New England Fall Conference

90

year. By the end of the decade, there were ten Regional Directors, still challenged with the need for help to get into 215 medical school campuses. Student work was still a priority.

Dr. Andrew Tsen, a cardiothoracic surgeon in Portland, Oregon, highlights the importance of student work from his own experience:

I entered medical school in the fall of 1984 like many first year initiates–fairly sure of my calling to medicine, but totally naïve and a little anxious about the experiences that lay ahead. College had been a heady time for me, and I grew deeper in my commitment to God. Medical school was different. Faith was more personal because there was little accountability. Faith also seemed more peripheral because it wasn't necessary for me to have it to succeed from the secular standpoint. Consequently, CMS became, for me, an integral part of navigating, spiritually intact, through those formative years.

The CMS group at the University of Kansas was just beginning to explode in numbers. The local campus ministry was also coupled to the national organization. We made sure that people joined, if nothing else, to get the Journal *and pertinent resource material.*

Our Regional Director at that time was Hal Habecker, who gently directed our effort to develop a successful campus ministry. Hal's vision of getting students to break out of the shell of their own campuses and see what the rest of the world was doing was pivotal. He got us to attend regional student leadership conferences, the national CMS meetings, and even the International Christian Medical & Dental Association meetings.

One of the highlights for me was our first national student conference in Dallas. Hal gave us the vision and empowerment to pull off the conference, which required months of planning, road trips to Dallas and even flights to England and Japan to see how other national student meetings were organized. It was a personal thrill to be rewarded with a Stetson cowboy hat at the end of the conference, but more importantly, to see the students gather to be challenged to live to make the difference in the midst of studies. That hat still sits through

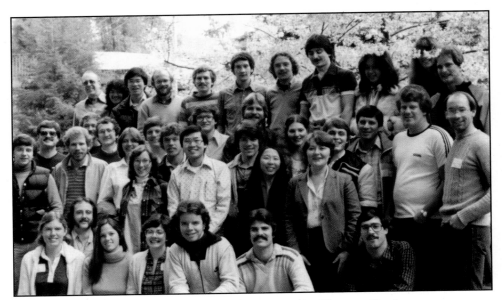

A Student Leadership Conference in Western Region.

residency, fellowship and private practice as a reminder of the importance of student ministry.

Today my wife, Ann, (whom I met through a MGM while we were both medical students) and I host the Oregon Health Sciences University medical school ministry at our home every other Wednesday evening, just like Dean Reeves did for me when I was a student in Kansas. In many ways, CMS came full circle for me. I want to keep the vision of how important this ministry is at a pivotal time in students' lives.

Perhaps there was not a lot of talk about mentoring of students, but it was going on. Dr. Jack Cooper of Dallas was an example. He was committed to discipling students at Southwestern Medical School, realizing that it was hard for them to keep their priorities straight during those demanding years. He took time to be with them at noon lunch meetings with Bible studies, he encouraged them to go on short-term mission trips, and he and his wife Nancy opened their home for Saturday morning breakfasts. It became a "home away from home" for some.

In 1988, the CMS name was changed to recognize more clearly whom the organization had represented for many years. Since 1984 a subtitle had been added "CMS—A Fellowship of Physicians and Dentists." But at the 1988 House of Delegates meeting in Seattle, the name became Christian Medical & Dental Society (CMDS).

Although the name changed, the ministry remained focused on changing lives. While in New Orleans for a society meeting, Hal Habecker met a member, Dr. Leo Happel, who was serving on the faculty of LSU Medical School. He asked Leo how he became involved with CMDS. Hal relates the story:

> Some years ago, a friend had sent Leo and his wife a gift Bible. Not being a Christian at that time, he was rather curious about the Bible, its place in his life, and what he was to do with it. At the same time, he noticed a little card on the bulletin board at the medical school that mentioned a weekly CMDS Bible study. He wondered if there was any connection between the two events.

> One day he bravely walked into the small room to find one of his best pupils, a freshman in physiology, Walter Larimore, teaching the Bible study. The conclusion of the story is that Walter, the first year medical student, had the privilege of leading his professor to faith in Christ several weeks later.

> Leo, looking me straight in the eye, said: "CMDS changed my life forever. Since that time, my wife and I have been privileged to lead over two dozen other couples to faith in Christ. Had it not been for Walter's bold faith and outreach in our lives, we might not be having this conversation tonight."

At the grassroots, local Chapters still were important and many new ones were formed, especially for fellowship. There also were an increased number or regional and local conferences.

In 1986, a National Convention was held in Dallas, following the House of Delegates meeting. The intention was that this would be the first such national convention to meet annually (others had been held sporadically before this). What has followed is a tradition to come together from all over the nation, to be challenged by speakers, to worship together, to encourage one another, and to share how God is at work. At the grass-roots, local Chapters still were important and many new ones were formed, especially for fellowship. There also were an increased number or regional and local conferences.

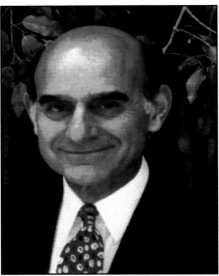

In May 1989, Dr. David Topazian, an Oral and Maxillofacial Surgeon and Associate Clinical Professor of Surgery at Yale, became President of CMDS, the first dental president for the Society. He led the organization into the next decade, when there would be new horizons to seek and challenges to meet.

David Topazian, D.D.S.,
CMDS President (1989-91)

* The booklet "Standards for Life," which contains all CMDA official statements on bioethical issues is available from CMDA by calling 1-888-231-2637.

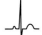

Chapter 8

Like a Rocket Ship on Its Way Up: The 1990s

$\mathcal{N}$ ot only was Dr. David Topazian the first dentist to become president of CMDS, he was also the first president who was, at the same time, a full-time foreign missionary. During his presidency, CMDS enjoyed a pronounced increase in its international influence. In response to concerns expressed by CMDS missionary members, the 1990 House of Delegates mandated that CMDS look into the problem of a shrinking pool of missionaries available for long-term services. A survey of mission agencies confirmed the belief of missionary members that the culprit was the high debt load incurred by most doctors during training.

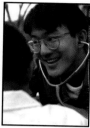

Educational debt was keeping many home.

As a result of this study, CMDS established a student debt relief fund, the goal of which was to place up to fifty missionaries on the mission field for long-term service. It was estimated that $10 million would be needed over time to accomplish this goal. The fund, which had its own Board of Trustees (reporting to the CMDS Board) would pay off a percentage of recipients' educational debt for each year served as long-term missionaries. In 1992, this student debt relief fund was independently incorporated as "Project MedSend," with the blessing of the CMDS Board.

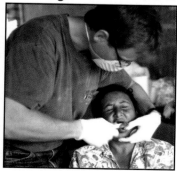

Project "MedSend" was established to help.

At about the same time, CMDS's Missionary Health Program (MHP) also incorporated separately from its parent organization, in this case to free CMDS from legal liability, while also allowing the Society to focus more on its main mission. This change came about as a result of a threatened lawsuit by one of the groups served by MHP. The suit was settled out of

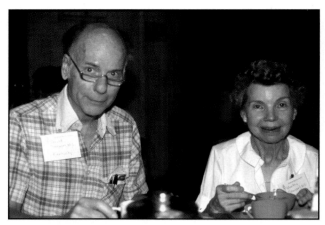

Drs. David and Martha Stewart

court in 1991, with MHP freeing money for the healthcare of the group's missionaries, while maintaining its own integrity, fiscally and otherwise.

In February 1990, the Continuing Medical and Dental Education (CMDE) conference in Kenya was attended by 285. At this conference, the first "David Stewart Memorial Lecture" was given by Dr. Ernie Steury. The lectureship, named in honor of one of the founders of the CMDE program, and established through many generous gifts in memory of Dr. Stewart, has provided honoraria, travel, and other expenses for each year's presenter since the inauguration of the series. *(Note: In 2002, the lecture was presented by Dr. Stewart's eighty-four-year-old widow, Dr. Martha Stewart.)*

The "Paul Tournier Institute" was established to address academic medical and dental issues in the context of the Christian community. The first meeting was held at the Georgetown University Conference Center, November 6-10, 1991. The conference, initiated by CMDS General Director Hal Habecker, Dr. Dale Mathews, and others, was chaired by Drs. David Allen and Edmund Pellegrino. Dr. Pellegrino's challenge was: "To be a physician is to be committed to a noble idea. To be a Christian physician is to add dimensions of inspiration and aspiration that elevate the ideal immeasurably. The Christian physician is called to imitate an ineffable model, an incarnate God whose own ministry was inseparable from healing."

Dr. Robert Kingsbury started his term as president in the fall of 1991. "I shall never forget the fervent prayer and 'laying on of hands' during the traditional president's breakfast," Kingsbury recalled. "I was assured that God would bless 'the little man with a big God.'" According to Dr. Kingsbury, one of the great blessings during his term as president was the time he spent traveling and working with Hal Habecker.

Following the death of *Journal* editor Sid Macaulay in 1991 (see chapter four) General Director Habecker filled in as editor of the *Journal* until 1992, when former CMDS New England regional director David B. Biebel, D. Min.—then editor of Focus on the Family's *Physician* magazine— returned to CMDS to edit the *Journal*, a role he continues to fulfill as this book is being prepared. Over the next few years, the *Journal* and the "News and Reports" were combined, the magazine's number of pages were increased, and a more practical, inspirational emphasis was adopted, with an expanded focus on the vision and activities of the organization.

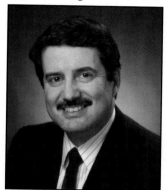

David Biebel, D.Min.

By the early 1990s, 40 percent of medical students were women and 1,300 CMDS members were women doctors. To more fully address the needs of these members, the CMDS board created an ad-hoc committee for Women in Medicine and Dentistry (WIMD). Dr.

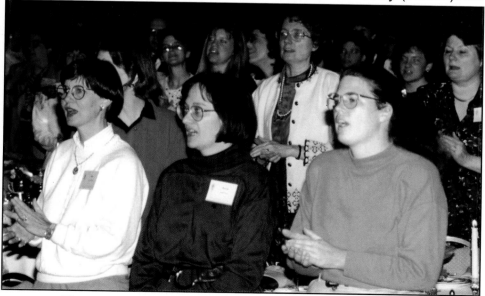

*Worship service the first Women in Medicine and Dentistry
National Conference (1994) — CMDS Journal archives*

Patti Francis did the first extensive survey of these members' interests and needs. She later passed the baton to Dr. Sally Knox who advanced the cause wonderfully. In April of 1992, Rev. Marti Ensign became the first director of this outreach, which provided resources directed toward women physicians and dentists, conferences to meet their specific needs, and a close-knit network to help them share and grow in Christ. In 1993, members of the WIMD Commission attended the American Medical Women's Association meeting, where many expressed an interest in CMDS. In April 1994, the first CMDS WIMD national convention was held.

One of the greatest challenges during Dr. Kingsbury's term was changing the function of the Board of Trustees from micromanagement to focusing on vision and strategic planning. The House of Delegates was also given the new tasks of functioning as the approval body for ethics statements and new Trustees.

One result of these changes was a new focus on improvement of benefits to members. CMDS began charging members lower conference registration fees than those paid by non-members. As a result of approval by the Accreditation Council for Continuing Medical Education) ACCME, CMDS began offering Category 1 CME credits at the organization's national conferences. Also, CMDS extended full membership eligibility to podiatrists, while adding a "friends" category for non-medical people with a heart for CMDS.

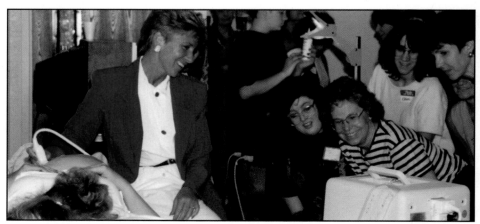

"Friend" of the Society, ultrasonographer Shari Richard, uses technology to show that the pre-born have fully human characteristics. — TCD Archives

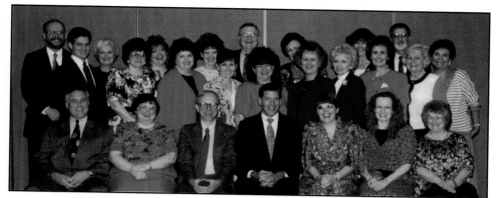

Richardson office personnel during Hal Habecker's tenure

Hal Habecker resigned as Executive Director of CMDS at the beginning of Dr. Robert Scheidt's presidency in September 1993. Hal was honored for his years of service at the 1994 national meeting. Hal became head pastor of a church in Dallas, Texas, where he still serves today. Hal's departing advice to Dr. Scheidt and the Board was to hire a physician to be the General Director. So the search began.

In Hal's absence, his executive secretary, Dorothy Rawles, fulfilled many of the duties of that office. She was nicknamed, "Pharaoh" because of how she very capably ran things. Dr. Scheidt said, "Dorothy was a one-woman army who procured meeting sites, organized the meetings, physically supervised the meeting rooms, equipment, banquets, and services at the hotels, and took all the minutes for the Trustees. I don't know how she did it. I'm just glad she did."

After a careful and prayerful process, the search committee, headed by Dr. Kingsbury, unanimously recommended that Dr. David Stevens become General Director (a position shortly thereafter renamed "Executive Director.") Dr. Stevens, a family physician, had worked overseas for eleven years as the medical director of Tenwek Hospital and was, at the time of his nomination, serving as the Executive Director of Samaritan's Purse.

Very soon after Dr. Stevens took office, he brought on Jonathan Imbody, M.A., as the Director of Advancement. Within a short time it

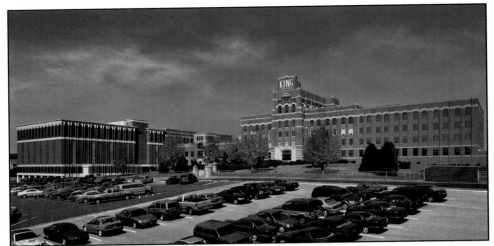
CMDS moved into the Bristol, Tennessee,
King Pharmaceuticals building in 1995.

became clear to the management and Trustees that the office space in Richardson, Texas, was not going to be adequate to support the organization's expanding vision, which included enhancing services to members and becoming the voice of Christian doctors in the exploding public debate over bioethical issues.

Almost as soon as the need for more space became apparent, it was met through the generosity of King Pharmaceuticals, Inc., in Bristol, Tennessee. The company had recently acquired ownership of an administration and manufacturing facility, which had previously been the international headquarters of Beecham Pharmaceuticals. The Gregory family, principle owners of King and Monarch Pharmaceuticals, offered CMDS a very low cost, 20-year lease of approximately 24,000 square feet of office and storage space. The Board spent a considerable amount of time debating the move and visiting the site. But in the end, the Board agreed that the advantages outweighed the negatives, and a decision to relocate was reached. For example, a feasibility study showed that CMDS would save more than a million dollars over the next five years by relocating to this facility. The TriCities area of Tennessee would provide an excellent environment, workforce, and low cost of living as compared with Richardson. The move would triple the useable office space, alleviating crowded conditions and allowing for much-needed growth.

The Richardson office personnel were offered a generous relocation package, but nearly all decided to take a severance package and stay in the Dallas area. Don Kencke, M.A., Director of Finance and Administration, temporarily relocated to Bristol for nearly two years, commuting monthly to Dallas to spend time with his family.

The facility in Dallas was sold to provide funds for severance packages and moving costs. New staff were hired in Bristol. Some traveled to Dallas for training over the six-month period prior to the move. The transition went smoothly with little interruption to member services.

During this time of major transitions, CMDS faced a difficult challenge from within. Those in charge of Medical Group Missions were not committed to the new leadership or the Board's vision for the ministry. Without the knowledge or consent of the administration or Board, this group incorporated a new organization. Attempts to resolve the conflict ultimately resulted in Christian mediation/arbitration. When it became apparent that the arbitration would go against the newly formed group, to foster a peaceful settlement and avoid further harm to the Lord's work, CMDS made the decision to transfer mission assets and a mailing list to the new work.

Shortly after the transition to Bristol, a placement service to match Christian doctors with Christian practices was launched. Within five months, the placement service had eleven signed contracts, twenty-five pending contracts, and twenty more in various stages of negotiation.

CMDS also started a new resource ministry called "Life & Health Resources." The first product was the "Prescribe A Resource." Using this resource, doctors could prescribe Christian resources for their patients by using a "prescription pad" designed for this purpose. These patients would then call CMDS to fill their "prescription." Since the inception of this pro-

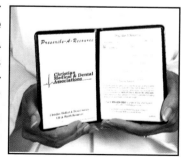

Prescribe A Resource

gram, thousands have acquired much-needed spiritual guidance through this outreach.

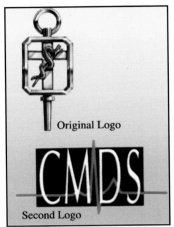

Original Logo

Second Logo

A new logo was designed for CMDS, and the name of the *Journal* became *Today's Christian Doctor*. New awards were also developed, including the Educator of the Year Award, the Missionary of the Year Award, and the President's Heritage award.

The Missionary of the Year award is presented to a missionary doctor who personifies love and passion for reaching unbelievers with the Gospel, an attitude of humility and service, demonstrates outstanding effectiveness in ministry, and inspires others to develop a heart for missions. Dr. Walter B. Hull was the first recipient.

The Educator of the Year award recognizes outstanding achievement in the area of medical or dental education. It is presented to a doctor who demonstrates an ability to instill in students a desire for professional excellence, lifelong learning, ethical integrity, unquestioned personal and professional integrity, and a commitment to biblical truth. Dr. William P. Wilson was the first recipient.

The President's Heritage Award is given to individuals who are non-members, who have contributed greatly to CMDS. Don Westra, J.D., was the initial recipient of this award. *(A complete listing of award recipients through the years may be found in the appendix.)*

In September 1994, Dr. Stevens and then Director of Advancement Jonathan Imbody cautiously considered a $500 expenditure for a press release announcing recent staff changes. They decided to do it and used the opportunity to represent CMDS as a broad movement of Christian doctors. The release, excerpted here, hit the wires—and made big news: "The medical community and those we serve must develop firm moral stances on the key bioethical issues of our day. . . . The Christian Medical & Dental Society stands in a unique position as a representative of thousands of Christian practitioners. . . ."

The Associated Press and PR Newswire picked up the piece, and it crossed the nation. Reporters arrived for interviews. Christian orga-

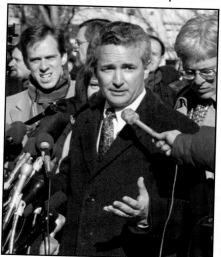

nizations called to express their solidarity. The National Council of Catholic Bishops requested qualified physicians to testify before the Supreme Court. At last, an organization of Christian professionals was addressing the perplexities of modern bioethical issues, and the nation took notice.

Since that first press release, constant demand for CMDS spokespersons indicates a tremendous hunger for a credible voice on complex ethical issues in both secular and Christian forums. Dr. Stevens esti-

Dr. David Stevens speaks to reporters.

mated that by the end of the 1990s he had spent over 1,000 hours speaking into microphones, whether on the steps of the U.S. Capitol, live on the "NBC Today" show, or in the studio producing *Christian Doctor's Digest* (*CDD*), CMDS's first audio magazine. These cassettes have been widely circulated by members among non-member colleagues, acquainting them with CMDS's mission, and driving significant membership increase.

For about a year and a half after the CMDS/MGM split, CMDS maintained a token mission program, utilizing a partnering program with likeminded mission programs and their leadership. Then the Board decided it was time to rebuild MGM. Dr. Stevens appointed Dr. Don Mullen as the new part-time director of MGM. Soon thereafter, the need for a new name became very evident in order to express clearly that a new missions outreach was being developed that would have an

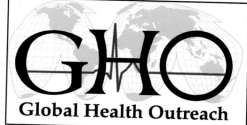

Global Health Outreach

emphasis on evangelism, leadership training and discipleship of participants, and partnering with local churches on the mission field. The name chosen was Global Health Outreach (GHO).

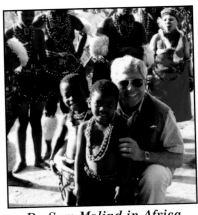

In 1997, Dr. Mullen stepped down as director to focus his energies on building a mission hospital in Greece. Dr. Sam Molind replaced him in 1998, moving to Bristol with his wife, Dorothy, leaving behind a very successful oral and

Dr. Sam Molind in Africa

maxillofacial surgical practice in Vermont. Sam was full of passion and energy, with a huge heart for missions. Through his leadership, GHO increased its number of trips per year, with half of the missions into Central and South America allowing for one-week missions in addition to the two-week opportunities in Zambia, Ethiopia, Ghana, Nigeria, Vietnam, Benin, Philippines, and Romania. A telephone affinity program was developed, with 10 percent of the proceeds returned to GHO. In its first year, the affinity program supplied $10,000 in income. That amount has increased to $40,000 per year, with an even greater potential for the future.

Soon after taking the reins of GHO, Dr. Molind began developing an intern-training program in short-term missions for missionology students at the local King College and Emmanuel College. Also, with the guidance and direction of Dave Bushong, CMDS Sight and Sound Director, footage was secured and photos acquired for a GHO promotional video, which has been very effective in recruitment and explaining the vision of GHO to others.

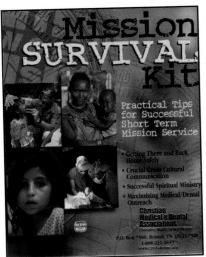

Misison Survival Kit

CMDS staff created an outline and audiotape series to help educate new participants about short-term medical missions. This "Missions Survival Kit" is now provided to every GHO participant. Also included in the orientation packet is a copy of the *Handbook of Medicine in Developing Countries*, by two of our members Drs. Catherine Wolf and Dennis Palmer.

In its first few years of existence, GHO forged mutually beneficial partnerships with key groups, including the Christian Pharmacists Fellowship International, the Nurses Christian Fellowship, the Fellowship of Christian Physician Assistants, and Prison Fellowship International.

In 1994, CMDS shifted paradigms in its approach to field ministries, as a community-based strategy was implemented. For years CMDS had employed a number of regional directors around the country who very capably carried out the CMDS ministry in their regions. These regional directors were expected to convey the vision of CMDS to the membership; train and disciple student leaders, campus advisors, and graduate leaders; be membership recruiters and fund-raisers; minister to the spiritual, emotional, and family needs of doctors; conduct conferences; and, periodically visit student and graduate chapters.

Now, the focus became grass roots leadership and development. The plan was to target certain areas (an "area" might be a campus, a city, or even a state) and to encourage groups of doctors to organize into local councils committed to being the owners and stewards of the ministry in their community—including raising all the funds needed to operate effectively.

In August 1994, Roger Matkin, D. Min., became CMDS's first area director. He had served effectively for years in San Antonio with the Texas Baptist Student Union and transitioned easily into his new role with

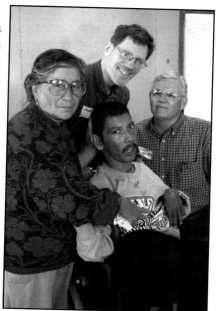

Roger Matkin, D. Min. (far right) and Donald Currie, M.D., caring for patients in Mexico

CMDS. Today, Roger leads a thriving ministry including Bible studies, noon luncheons, and monthly medical/dental mission trips into Mexico with graduates and students.

In June 1998, Dale Holloway, Ph.D., became the first full-time director of Community Based Ministries (CBM). Currently the organization has nine area directors,* while continuing to promote the concept of CBM, nationwide. In addition to full-time area directors, there are also several associate staff who minister part-time on various campuses.

Meanwhile, the need for regional directors has not diminished. Indeed, the regional directors* play a crucial administrative role in the new community-based approach to ministry, with much of their energy focused on establishing local councils.

In June 1999, Ron Brown, M.A., joined the GHO staff as Associate Director. Ron came from a pastoral background, with administrative experience. At about that same time, Mr. and Mrs. Joe Luce gave GHO a 38-foot-long prototype "Wonderlodge" built by Blue Bird Corporation. Joe spent many hours working on the Wonderlodge with Donnie Hobbs to prepare it for its new mission as a Mobile

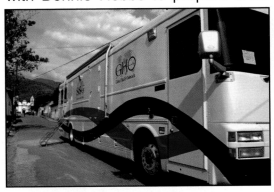
GHO's Mobile Medical Unit

Medical Unit (MMU) that would function as part of the "Caravan of Hope" for medical ministry in Honduras. The shell of the MMU was finished and equipped through approximately $200,000 in donations from members and friends. It contained a state-of-the-art lab designed and installed by Ed Bos, president of World Wide Labs, a surgical suite, and X-ray capabilities. The summer 2000 issue of *Today's Christian Doctor* featured the MMU's "Maiden Voyage" to Jesus de Otoro, Honduras.

An effective outreach was developed in Honduras with the able leadership of Dan and Jessica Eberhard, who served as GHO missionaries to Honduras until 2000. Their trailblazing efforts and organization established the GHO ministry in Honduras as a spiritual ministry using medicine and dentistry as a conduit for the Gospel, and bringing evangelical churches together to impact their communities for Christ.

On another "outreach" front, a membership survey had confirmed that, above all else, members valued CMDS as their national voice. The vision was defined: *to speak out, representing and equipping members to change the heart of healthcare.* As CMDS strengthened ties to fellow national Christian organizations, opportunities arose across the Christian media. For example, the American Family Association requested 100 yearly public service announcements on health and bioethics for broadcast on their radio network.

By the time Oregon faced its second referendum to legalize physician-assisted suicide in 1997, CMDS was working to equip and educate members to fight the dangerous bill. Although "Measure 51" passed, making Oregon the first state to sanction the lethal use of doctors' resources, CMDS learned valuable lessons through the experience and determined to halt the "right-to-die" momentum. "We realized that we had to fight the battle on many levels," Dr. Stevens said.

A year later, Michigan voters faced a similar referendum to legalize physician-assisted suicide. But this time, CMDS strategized to work through physicians, churches, medical school chapters, and statewide media. Members were mobilized and armed with videos, books, and teaching materials from the "Battle for Life" kits to educate their churches and colleagues. The CMDS campaign swept through Michigan in a week—with Dr. Stevens speaking at each medical school, talking to healthcare groups, and making media appearances. Stevens and the CMDS media team

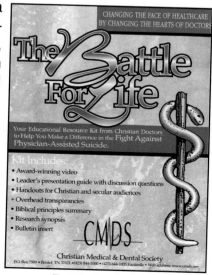

Battle for Life kit

developed a twenty-minute "Chat With Your Family Doctor" video on physician-assisted suicide, offered to churches. Over 400 churches requested the program, airing CMDS's message to thousands of parishioners on the Sunday before the vote.

CMDS Midwestern Regional Director Allan Harmer, Th.M., networked with local members, identifying a bureau of spokespersons to speak in area churches. A special edition of "Healthwise" public service announcements on physician-assisted suicide was aired on Christian radio across the state. And, using a model letter from CMDS, physicians notified their patients of their commitment to life-affirming care and opposition to physician-assisted suicide.

CMDS was determined to take the warning against physician-assisted suicide into every home across the state, despite the fact that a single thirty-second ad on prime time TV can cost more than $50,000. Media and Public Relations Coordinator Annemarie Dugan had just come to CMDS from the television newsroom. She recognized that CMDS had the elements to make great news—doctors, patients, and a vested interest in opposing the referendum. An objective "third person" report on the opinions and activities of CMDS physicians could be aired as local news. So Dugan initiated the first CMDS video news release.

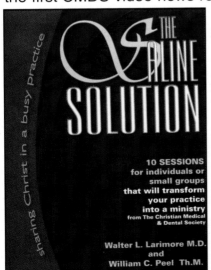

The Saline Solution video series

CMDS members had also indicated their desire for resources to enable evangelism and spiritual growth. *The Saline Solution* was developed by William Peel, Th.M., and Dr. Walt Larimore. By the end of the decade, this conference and video series had taught more than 6,000 people how to share their faith in their practice. Peel also produced the student study guidebook, *Living in the Lab Without Smelling Like a Cadaver*, published in 1999 by CMDS's "Paul Tournier Institute" division, of which Peel was director at the time. This was the first of a new series of books produced in-house to address specific membership needs and concerns.

During the 1990s, with the escalation of medical malpractice litigations, CMDS received an ever-increasing number of calls from members requesting spiritual support and other resources because they had been sued. In response to this need, the Medical Malpractice Ministry (3M) was established. The first meeting of the new Commission that would oversee this ministry's development was held in 1998. In his portion of the 1999 CMDS Annual Report, published in *Today's Christian Doctor* (Winter 1999), Commission chair Curtis E. Harris, M.D., J.D., reported that this outreach effort of CMDS had received eighty calls during the prior year. "All of the callers requested the free malpractice resource kit," Curtis reported, "twenty-two percent requested phone counseling with a member of the 3M Commission; and, 18 percent borrowed the video entitled 'Malpractice: A Survival Guide for Physicians and Their Families.'"

In 1999, CMDS opened an office in Washington, D.C., staffed by Jonathan Imbody. "It's amazing how dependent representatives, senators, and others are on individual groups for their information," Dr. Stevens explained. "We want to be a source of expert informa-

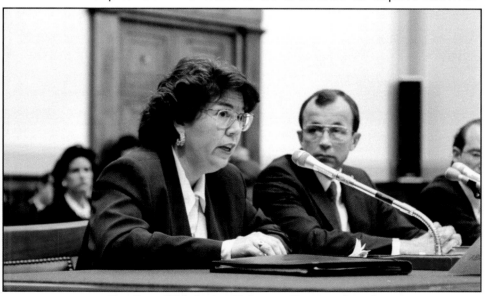

Dr. Jean Wright testifying at Congressional
"Partial-birth" Abortion Hearing

tion that our legislators can trust. On Capitol Hill, CMDS will be available—for Senate hearings, emergency press conferences, media networking, and consultation with lawmakers."

As a result of all these changes and the development of new ministries in response to the needs and desires of Society members, by the end of the twentieth century CMDS was like a rocket ship on its way up!

The Placement Service had linked hundreds of doctors and other healthcare professionals with practices that shared their values. It had developed a seminar for medical students entitled, "Preparing the Way: A Guide to Finding Your First Practice."

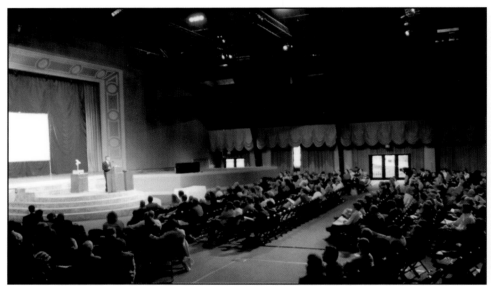

This conference, jointly sponsored by CMDS and Focus on the Family, was attended by hundreds of physicians and spouses.

Life & Health Resources had fulfilled thousands of requests for books, audio tapes, videotapes, and other resources. CMDS meetings had seen dramatically increased attendance, partly due to the opportunity to earn Continuing Education credits. In 1999 alone, more than 3,600 individuals registered for CMDS's meetings.

CMDS was continuing to distribute its forty-page *SCAN*—a monthly survey of medical/dental articles of special interest to missionary doctors working overseas, edited by Dr. Richard Roach with the able

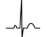

assistance of Associate Editor Renee Hyatt—to approximately 1,000 recipients worldwide.

Evangelism had grown through programs like *The Saline Solution* series. GHO had expanded its outreach to over thirty trips per year, while hiring full-time Honduras staff to run the MMU ministry. "CMDS Healthwise" radio spots were being aired on 600 stations nationwide, educating the public about health-related issues as well as the existence of this special group of doctors. CMDS was being barraged with media requests for qualified spokespersons for interviews.

Discipleship had reached new heights, with CMDS representation on more than ninety percent of medical and dental school campuses. The Singles Ministry, with the help of long-time regional director Michael McLaughlin, was networking over 4,000 single members, while providing special activities and avenues of service for them.

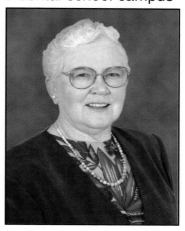

The Women in Medicine & Dentistry ministry was continuing to grow and minister to women physicians and dentists, through the leadership of the new ministry director, Harriet Askew, and the enthusiastic help of the WIMD Commission.

Dorthy Barbo, M.D.,
CMDS President (1997-99)

Other Commissions also continued to increase their outreach and effectiveness as the needs of medical and dental professionals were identified. For example, the Ethics Commission continued to develop statements addressing crucial bioethical issues, while also developing a bioethics consultation service. The Marriage and Family Commission sponsored nine Marriage Enrichment Conferences in 1999, providing 110 doctors and their spouses with counsel, support, and an opportunity to strengthen their marriage vows.

The COIMEA Commission continued to expand its efforts, worldwide, offering educational physicians and dentists an opportunity to witness through teaching. The Domestic Missions Commission developed and implemented a strategy to involve more physicians and dentists in caring for the underserved. The 3M Commission focused on training more counselors as the number of calls increased. The CMDE Commission heard from an ever-increasing

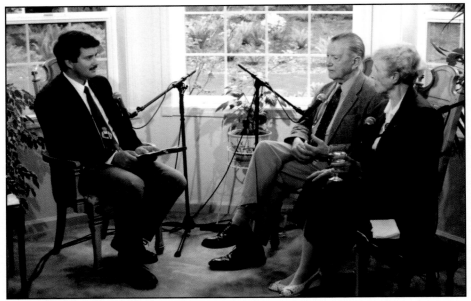

A videotaped interview of Drs. Paul and Margaret Brand, "A Single Vision," covers: Putting the Joy Back in Medicine; What is Success?; Integrating Faith & Medicine; The Doctor-Patient Relationship; and, Building a Marriage Relationship That Lasts.

number of missionary doctors and others wishing to participate in the CMDE programs.

By serving as the voice of Christian doctors and providing resources and opportunities for evangelism, discipleship, networking, and service, CMDS had, during the 1990s, become a well-coordinated, multi-faceted effort to change the face of healthcare. Membership had grown to 14,200 with a 92 percent retention rate. The annual budget topped $6 million, yet the organization finished the 1999 fiscal year in the black and with adequate reserves to face an uncertain future.

*A complete listing of current field staff can be found in the appendix.

Chapter 9

Carrying the Torch into the New Millennium

*Y*2K brought many fresh, new ideas and initiatives for CMDS. In January 2000, the Board appointed a strategic planning committee to work with Dr. David Stevens and TEAM Resources of Atlanta, Georgia, to establish a five-year plan. The process was long, intense, and laborious, but very effective. The committee came out of the strategic planning

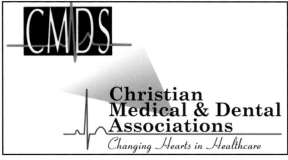

CMDS and CMDA logos

process renewed, with a new passion for the future of the organization. From the strategic planning session, leadership came away with a new mission statement, a vision for the future, core values,[1] defined ministries, goals and benchmarks, strategies, and a new name to guide it into the first part of the 21st century.

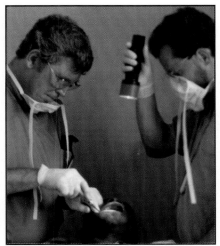

"CMDA" indicates a greater emphasis on dental members.

As a result of the new strategic plan, CMDS became the Christian Medical & Dental Associations (CMDA), because "CMDS" had become difficult to use, especially as the organization increasingly spoke for its members on bioethical issues. The media couldn't remember "CMDS" or butchered it in interviews. Some questioned why a "dental" organization was addressing ethical issues. The name change also presented a new opportunity to specifically address the needs of dental members, through a dental division with a full-time dental director. Also, changing the name to "Associations" allowed CMDA to use "Christian Medical Association" when addressing a medical or media audience and "Christian Dental Association" when describing its dental outreach.

CMDA's five areas of ministry were clearly defined—evangelism, discipleship, service, resources, and voice. The Board and management would use key indicators in these five areas of ministry to check the "pulse" of the organization on a regular basis.

Another part of the strategic plan was the Board's decision to purchase more than fifty acres of beautiful land near Bristol as a future building site. After five years of being located in the King Pharmaceutical building, staff and ministries had more than doubled, and CMDA was "bursting at the seams!" The $10 million capital campaign was launched by a $3 million gift from donors who wished to remain anonymous.

Past Presidents Drs. Bob Agnew and Dorothy Barbo became co-chairs of the capital campaign. Working with consultants out of Atlanta, they began the "silent phase" of the campaign for solicitation of major gifts. Through the end of 2001, the effort had raised more than half of its goal, with the public phase of the campaign scheduled to begin during the spring of 2002. The campaign not only included constructing a new 52,000 sqare-foot headquarters for

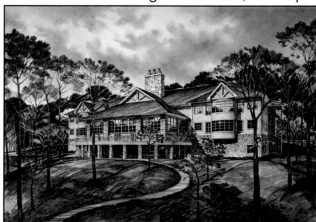

CMDA, but also providing new capabilities for enhanced ministry and growth – such as a satellite link for national TV media interviews, storage for equipment and medicines for medical mission outreach, and more room for expanding current ministries. The new

New CMDA headquarters in Bristol, Tennessee

headquarter's design also included a conference space for 250 people for regional conferences and leadership training.

Before Bill Peel resigned as the director of the Paul Tournier Institute in June 2000 to take a church pastoral position, he had supervised the production of a video version of The Saline Solution conference for small group use. After his resignation, Bill continued to teach Saline Solution conferences and work with the video series. By September 2000, over eight hundred copies of the video series had been purchased. Also, numerous international organizations 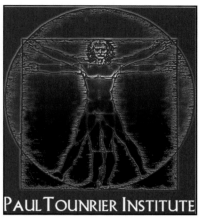 had contacted CMDA for permission to translate the series into other languages, and to host conferences internationally.

One new initiative that continued into the new millennium was called "The Future of Medicine." The first meeting had been held in late 1999. Following this meeting, CMDA member Dr. Jean Wright became the driving force behind the initiative to provide alternative healthcare delivery options for the Christian community. Dr. Wright resigned from her full-time practice to devote herself to the Future of Medicine initiative, meeting with other healthcare leaders, researching healthcare information, developing new ideas, and trying to sell those ideas to other organizations.

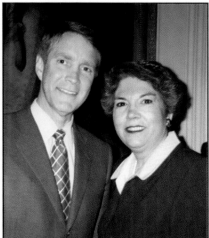

Tennessee Senator Dr. Bill Frist meets Dr. Jean Wright during one of her visits to Washington, D.C.

In 2000, Rev. Marti Ensign retired from the leadership of Women in Medicine & Dentistry (WIMD). She was recognized for her faithful service at the 2000 National Convention. Harriet Askew became the new director of the WIMD, and has been working diligently with the commission since.

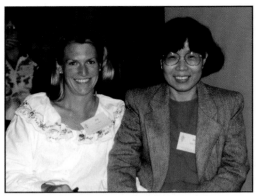

The WIMD outreach provides opportunities for fellowship and support.

As a need for more guidance for commissions became evident, Dr. Stevens developed a commission handbook, which has been a great tool to aid chairpersons in their leadership role. The booklet lays out the structure of commissions, how they work with the home office, and procedures for all aspects of their ministry.

In November 2000, CMDA jointly sponsored and spearheaded an effort to bring a wide variety of ministries together for an annual medical missions conference with Southeast Christian Church in Louisville, Kentucky. This meeting, with forty workshops packed into a two-day conference, was attended by 800 participants and attracted exhibitors from around the world. The goal of the conference was to provide a place for recruiting the next generation of healthcare missionaries and a forum for networking, training and strategizing how to better carry out the Great Commission.

CMDA and Zondervan Publishing Corporation entered into a joint agreement in late 1999 to co-publish a series of lay-level books that are "medically reliable and biblically sound." The first book in this series, released in April 2001, was *Jesus, MD: A Doctor Looks at the Great Physician* by David Stevens, M.D., with Gregg Lewis. The second title, *Alternative Medicine: The Christian Handbook*, written by Walt Larimore, M.D., and Donal O'Mathuna, Ph.D.,

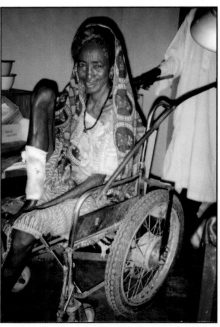

Supporting long- and short-term missions work is still a high priority of CMDA.
—*TCD Archives,*
Courtesy of Dr. & Mrs. Harold Adolph

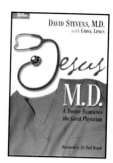
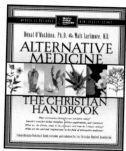
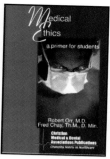
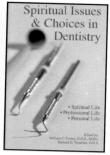

was also released in 2001. The goal is to jointly publish, over a five-year period, twenty or more books with a distinctly Christian approach to a wide range of issues from breast cancer to depression.

Also released in 2001 were two new books published "in house" by the Paul Tournier Institute division of CMDA. These books, aimed specifically at members' interests and needs were: *Medical Ethics: A Primer for Students*, by Robert D. Orr, M.D., and Fred Chay, D. Min., and *Spiritual Issues and Choices in Dentistry*, edited by William C. Forbes, D.D.S., M.Div., and Richard G. Topazian, D.D.S.

Through the generosity of a CMDA member, the "Ernest Steury, M.D., Scholarship Fund" was established in January 2001. This fund provides significant tuition assistance for four years to a medical student who is committed to a career in foreign or domestic medical missions. Scott Lawrence, previous Northeast Regional Director of CMDA, was the first recipient of this award.

After much hard work, GHO's Mobile Medical Unit (MMU) was put into service the week before Easter 2000, when a team of twenty-five, went to help the people of Jesus de Otoro, Honduras. The team worked in a school with the bus parked just outside the gate on the street. Ed Bos, of World Wide Lab Improvement, who had set up the MMU's lab, went on the trip to ensure that the equipment functioned well. The X-ray equipment was a godsend because of the high incidence of TB in the area. The team did a number of minor surgeries, including repairing a severely lacerated toe that a boy had caught in a bicycle spoke. On one afternoon, the team did home visits to disabled children and shut-ins. In one home, Dr. Stevens, the team leader, found a woman writhing in pain. She had a gangrenous foot

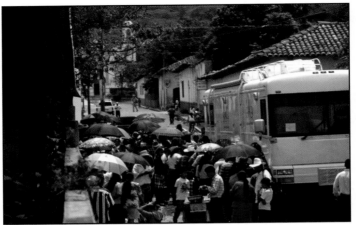
The Mobile Medical Unit in action

that needed to be amputated. He started her on antibiotics and fluids and the team gave the money necessary to have surgery done at a hospital some distance away. Without the team's help, this woman would have died. In all, the team saw and shared the Gospel with more than 1,800 patients.

By 2001, GHO's annual schedule had expanded to thirty trips per year. It had become one of the finest short-term medical/dental mission experiences available. A formal leadership training program with on-the-field mentoring had been established. The outreach was providing mandatory professional and spiritual leadership training for its team leaders, including field staff that might participate. A GHO leadership manual—provided to each team leader—outlined expectations, policies and procedures, limitations, and other valuable information. Trips focused first on spiritually impacting each participant, secondly on spiritually impacting the community, and thirdly on strengthening local churches and pastors. Months before each trip, GHO staff in Honduras visited prospective sites, located and trained pastors and volunteers, met with government officials, and secured local translators. Each team member had opportunities to witness in song, word, and deed with the assurance that the hundreds that came to Christ on each trip would be nurtured in their newfound faith in a local church body. In 2001, close to 10,000 people accepted Christ through GHO trips and ninety percent of them were in ongoing discipleship groups.

Much of the success of GHO could be attributed to excellent leadership in the U.S. and the CMDA staff in Central America, Ricardo Castro and Dr. Brent Hambrick.

The added trips and increasing number of applicants were a blessing, yet a strain on the staff. When budget constraints kept GHO from hiring additional personnel to keep up with the demand, Dorothy Molind, wife of GHO Director Sam Molind, organized a team of local volunteers to send out mailings, stock medicines, pull supplies, and perform many other tasks.

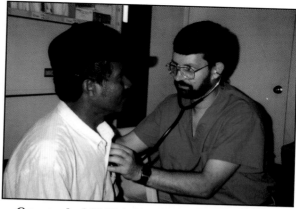

One goal of CMDA Short-term missions is to change the hearts of participants. Dr. David Drozek became a full-time missionary in Honduras after a short-term mission.
(See the Summer 2001 issue, Today's Christian Doctor)

Since its inception, CMDA's community-based ministry (CBM) had been mobilizing and equipping local doctors to minister to the spiritual needs of students and colleagues. As one of many possible examples, Midwest Regional Director Allan Harmer received a call from Annemarie Daly, M.D., who wanted to know what CMDA was doing in Detroit. Allan explained that he had been praying for God to raise up a key doctor who would help lead a new movement there. Annemarie said that just the night before at her church's mission conference, she had offered herself to be used by the Lord. However, she wondered how He could use a mother of five in foreign missions. But as Allan continued to share CMDA's vision, Annemarie realized the Lord did, indeed, have a plan for her—in Detroit. She immediately went to work recruiting doctors and formed a CMDA local council. In just a short time, that ministry took off and an associate staff person was hired to give direction to the new effort. In 2001, the CBM division established an online mentoring service for residents, linking practicing members, who wished to mentor, with residents via the CMDA Web site. The plan was that after fourth-year students received their residency match, they would be able to find a mentor in the city of their residency. CBM's expectation is that this service, will, over time, meet a distinct need for residents.

During the November 2000 CMDA/Focus on the Family joint conference, Drs. Paul and Margaret Brand were presented with the first CMDA "Great Physician" award. This award was given because of their work of touching the untouchable, restoring the disfigured, and offering eternal hope for impoverished souls in India and around the world, where Paul had specialized in hand reconstruction with lepers and Margaret had used her ophthalmology skills to prevent blindness.

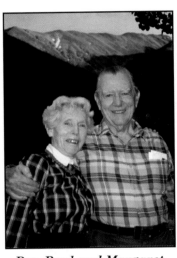

Drs. Paul and Margaret Brand

On December 31, 2000, Dr. Bob and Marian Schindler retired from being co-administrators of the COIMEA. The Spring 2001 issue of *Today's Christian Doctor* featured a "Thank You Tribute" written by Dr. Jeff Barrows, current COIMEA assistant administrator, acknowledging their development, on-going work, and passion for COIMEA. Echoing the experience of many others through the years, Dr. Neal Smith stated, "Bob encouraged me to go behind the Iron Curtain and that I could have an impact. He was right. I was honored to be used by God, and Bob and Marian were His instruments."

On March 8, 2001, the Christian Medical Association joined in a lawsuit filed on behalf of parents of adopted human embryos, an embryo adoption agency, research scientists, and others against the National Institutes of Health (NIH). The suit's aim was to require the NIH to obey the congressional ban on funding research involving the destruction of human embryos. This lawsuit propelled CMDA into the limelight on the embryonic stem cell issue and created opportunities for Michael West of Advanced Cell Technologies and others on CNN and other major media outlets. The stipulations in the lawsuit were agreed to by NIH late in 2001.

Two days before the Board was scheduled to meet in Albuquerque, N.M., in September 2001, terrorist attacks occurred in N.Y., Washington, and Pennsylvania. CMDA cancelled the Board meeting

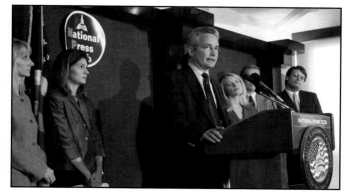

Dr. Stevens explains CMDA et al v. NIH lawsuit at press conference.

and immediately contacted members who were qualified counselors to link them to churches and other outreaches to provide free counseling to the victims of this terrible tragedy.

One reason CMDA's response time to this crisis was so brief was the many improvements made in the Member Services division during the previous several years. By 2001, the database had been fully computerized and updated. New invoicing techniques had been implemented. Recruitment of new members had been enhanced, bringing membership to 15,454 by the end of 2001.

CMDA had also launched a new Web site: http://www.cmdahome.org. In one ten-month period, the site had been visited 750,000 times. The most popular components of the Web site were membership, the resources shopping area, the "News & Views" electronic newsletter, and the Washington Bureau section—which kept members updated on fast-breaking policy and ethics news. In addition, member services also had created a twenty-eight-page booklet called the "Guide to Member Services" summarizing the many ministries of CMDA.

By its seventieth anniversary, CMDA had enhanced communication with its members through *Today's Christian Doctor* magazine and the acclaimed *Christian Doctor's Digest* audio series. *The Saline Solution* conference had trained over 10,000 participants, and many more had learned the program's principles through a video/workbook series. CMDA's growth and strong retention rate were in part the result of addressing the felt needs of its members, including job placement assistance, bioethics consultation, and support for those going through the agony of malpractice litigation. CMDA had deepened and broadened its ministry through adopting a community-

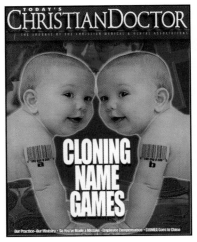

TODAY'S
CHRISTIAN DOCTOR
THE JOURNAL OF THE CHRISTIAN MEDICAL & DENTAL ASSOCIATIONS

CLONING
NAME
GAMES

a   b

Our Practice—Our Ministry • So You've Made a Mistake • Employee Compensation • CMDA Goes to China

based philosophy of ministry. As a result, by the end of 2001, the number of campus field staff had more than tripled. The organization had revamped and refocused its short-term mission outreach. It had set up a forward operations base in Central America to facilitate logistics and relationships and the most effective use of the MMU in the field. Strategic alliances with Focus on the Family, Prison Fellowship International, the Center for Bioethics and Human Dignity, and many other groups had increased CMDA's influence and impact.

CMDA had taken its ethical statements off the shelf and become a compelling voice on behalf of its members on bioethics and healthcare issues in the public arena. Through a joint publishing agreement with Zondervan Corporation, by airing public service announcements on 600 stations, conducting grass roots campaigns to defeat euthanasia referendums, giving four hundred media interviews a year, providing congressional testimony, and establishing a Washington, D.C., office, CMDA was impacting the course of healthcare in America, perhaps far more than its founders had ever imagined possible.

Yet the question remained: What does the future hold for medicine and dentistry? And the challenge remained: How can CMDA better motivate, train, and equip Christians in healthcare for service in the future? CMDA's CEO Dr. David Stevens offered the following analysis, and ten "marching orders" for the future:

There will be constant and profound changes in healthcare for the foreseeable future, driven by new technology, out-of-control costs, litigation, changes in healthcare delivery, and increasing government involvement. Just as, in 1931, CMDA's founders couldn't fully envision what would happen in medicine over the next seven decades, we can only imagine what lies ahead. We see things like regenerative medicine, genetic manipulation, computerization,

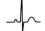

robotic surgery, and escalating costs and wonder where they will take us. We see trust—at the center of the doctor-patient relationship—disintegrating. We see secular pluralism eroding traditional values and Hippocratic medicine.

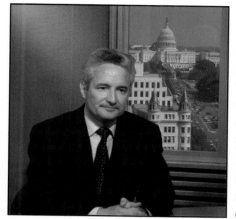
Dr. Stevens in Washington

In just the past few years, ethical debate has shifted from abortion to physician assisted suicide, destructive embryonic stem cell research, cloning, fetal harvesting, and ethical issues flowing from the human genome project. Looking down the road it is easy to see the oncoming headlights of gender selection, nanotechnology, designer babies, germ cell line manipulation, euthanasia, xenotransplantation, genetic determinism, and human reproductive cloning. And there is no doubt that other ethical issues will arise that we can't imagine now.

As I see it, God has raised up and prepared CMDA for such a time as this—to battle for truth in His name. And as I've thought about these issues in relation to CMDA, I can discern ten marching orders that God would give us in the days ahead:

1. We must provide excellent basic training. We will lose the war by attrition if we don't insure that new recruits into the medical and dental professions are firmly grounded in Christ and the truth of the Word of God. CMDA must strive for a vibrant and comprehensive ministry on every medical and dental school campus in the United States. Using our community based ministry approach, our goal will be to motivate and train local Christian doctors to make discipling students a priority—organizing councils in the vicinity of every campus.

2. We must reaffirm our individual orders. Doctors are leaving medicine in large numbers as conditions worsen. Christian doctors must not join this retreat but instead reaffirm that God has called us to minister through healthcare. Our confidence that God Himself has commissioned us will strengthen us to not grow weary in well doing and to follow our marching orders.

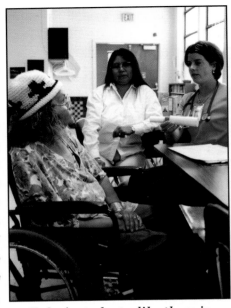

3. We must equip our minds for the battles ahead. The enemy is skillful and difficult to defeat. He is using new weapons of mass destruction from the media to the Internet to sway minds and hearts on ethical, moral, and policy issues. CMDA is committed to equipping our members with the weapons of apologetics, ethics, compelling data, and new battle strategies. For example, we are working on DVDs containing a wealth of resources – Power Point

Today's students, like those in CMDA's earliest days, want to serve as they learn.
—Courtesy, Summer Medical Institute Northwest 2000 (see TCD, Summer 2001)

presentations, handouts, bulletin inserts, videos, audio tapes, sample letters, biblical references, sound bites, and much more.

4. We must improve our communication. We are looking for better ways to provide the information that members need and want in order to keep abreast of current events and to provide this critical

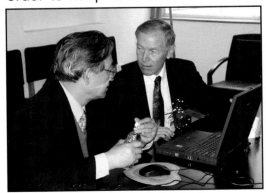

information on a timely basis. To this end we are reorganizing our Web site, revamping our "News & Views" format, and expanding our number of *Christian Doctor's Digests.* Soon we will be moving to a totally electronic communication system with students— the format they want. This will let us make student memberships free, giving them access

Technology is the key to education and communication. Shown is Dr. Douglas W. Soderdahl, on a 2001 COIMEA trip to China, with his "ever present" laptop.

to *Christian Doctor's Digest* and *Today's Christian Doctor* magazine via the Internet.

Our communication to the church and media must also improve. CMDA's new headquarters will contain modern TV and radio studios with a satellite earth station to link directly to networks. Members and staff will be available on short notice for major TV talk and news shows. We plan to produce and upload video news releases on a host of important topics for local TV news shows across the country. A radio program is on the drawing board so that we can equip the church on important health and ethical issues.

5. We must continue to forge strategic alliances. We can't win this war alone. We have already been working with other professional organizations such as Christian Pharmacy Fellowship, the Fellowship of Christian Physician Assistants, Focus on the Family, the Christian Legal Society, Nurses Christian Fellowship, and the Center for Bioethics and Human Dignity. We have been offering our expertise and that of our members to the government, prolife groups in Washington, D.C., and churches across the country. We want to expand these strategic alliances because there is strength in numbers.

6. We must amplify our firepower by expanding our membership. We estimate there are 75,000 to 100,000 doctors in the U.S. who should be in CMDA. We want to expand our membership to 30,000 by 2007. We hope to be able to reduce our dues to lower the financial barrier to joining. Already we have a pay-as-you-can policy that needs to be more widely known. To lower dues, we must strengthen our financial position. Imagine our impact if CMDA were larger than ACOG, the AFFP, other specialty organizations, or even the AMA?

7. We must gain the high ground. That is why I have been so excited to see our members accepting positions at NIH, HHS, the CDC, and other places in government. It is thrilling to see Christian physicians in Congress and taking roles in their specialty groups. We must gain the high ground if we are going to win battles.

8. We must strengthen our supply lines. We could do so much if we just had the funds. We need to add a physician ethicist to specifically work on getting articles into major journals and to write "white papers" for Congress. We need a staff of research associates constantly combing the research for data "ammunition" useful to our side. We need to add a dentist to strengthen our outreach to dental campuses and to produce dental resources. This, we believe, would quadruple our dental membership. We need more staff in our donor services department to help members with estate planning and to approach foundations for grants. Funds are needed for resource and media production. Wars cost money and usually the side with the most resources wins.

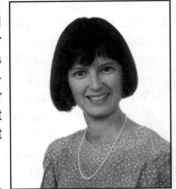

Dr. Clydette Powell, Medical Officer, Global Tuberculosis programs, U.S. Agency for International Development

9. We must increasingly go on the offensive. Too often our energies have been consumed by fighting a defensive war as we see our traditional values and territories attacked, when the best defense in our situation may be a stronger offense. Christian doctors must establish new strategies and set the agenda to which others will respond. Dr. David Larson, at the National Institute of Healthcare Research (renamed in 2001, the "International Center for the Integration of Health & Spirituality") did this masterfully by demonstrating the link between faith and health. Other CMDA members, including Dr. Harold Koenig, author of *The Healing Connection*, and founder and director of Duke University's Center for the Study of Religion/Spirituality and Health and Dr. Dale Matthews, author of *The Faith Factor* have also contributed to this area of study. CMDA has used this research to teach Christian doctors how to meet the spiritual needs of their patients. To go on the offensive in other areas, I'm convinced that CMDA must be involved in research, curriculum development, and resource production. We must mobilize, network, and motivate our troops to focus on specific objectives, while providing them the ammunition they need.

10. We must improve our morale. As I talk to members, I often find discouraged and demoralized soldiers who have, at least temporarily, forgotten whose side we are on. Our commander-in-chief is the Lord Himself. Archangels serve at our side. And, we should derive courage because we already know the final outcome of the war. Yet our strength can only be maintained through daily rations of prayer, time in the Scriptures, and regular fellowship with our comrades in arms. Thankfully, in the end our performance will be

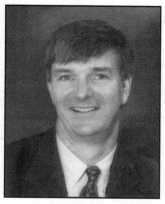

Dr. David Larson

judged not by individual skirmishes won or lost, but by whether or not we were faithful.

Without doubt, CMDA made such enormous strides in its first seventy years because of the faithfulness of thousands of members and scores of leaders whose perseverance and courage set the standard for us. Now, it's our turn to boldly advance the cause. And as each of us enters the fray, CMDA will be there to motivate, train, encourage, equip, and provide the resources needed as we continue to (if I may paraphrase the Apostle Paul): "...conduct [ourselves] in a manner worthy of the gospel of Christ...standing firm in one spirit, with one mind striving together for the faith of the gospel; in no way alarmed by [our] opponents...which is a sign of destruction for them, but of salvation for [us], and that, too, from God" (Philippians 1:27-28, NASB).

1. The CMDA mission, vision, and core values statements are found in the appendix.

128

Appendix

CMDA Vision Statement

Transforming tens of thousands of doctors to change their world as they:
1. bring people to Christ
2. raise up the next generation of Christian doctors
3. sacrificially serve those in need
4. integrate their faith into their practice
5. speak out as the trusted voice on bioethics to our culture

CMDA Mission Statement

Christian Medical & Dental Association exists to motivate, educate, and equip Christian physicians and dentists to glorify God:
- by living out the character of Christ in their homes, practices, and around the world;
- by pursuing professional competence and Christ-like compassion in their daily work;
- by influencing their families, colleagues, and patients toward a right relationship with Jesus Christ;
- by advancing Biblical principles in bioethics and health to the church and society.

CMDA Core Values

We strive to fulfill our mission by commitment to be:

- **Christ-like**
  Your attitude should be the same as that of Christ Jesus: Philippians 2:5
- **Controlled by the Holy Spirit**
  But when he, the Spirit of truth, comes, he will guide you into all truth. He will not speak on his own; he will speak only what he hears, and he will tell you what is yet to come. He will bring glory to me by taking from what is mine and making it known to you. John 16:13&14
- **Committed to Scripture**
  Your word is a lamp to my feet and a light for my path. Psalm 119:105
- **Communing in Prayer**
  And pray in the Spirit on all occasions with all kinds of prayers and requests. With this in mind, be alert and always keep on praying for all the saints. Ephesians 6:18
- **Compassionate**
  "A new command I give you: Love one another. As I have loved you, so you must love one another. By this all men will know that you are my disciples, if you love one another." John 13:34&35
- **Competent**
  In the same way, let your light shine before men, that they may see your good deeds and praise your Father in heaven. Matthew 15:16

- **Courageous**
  For God did not give us a spirit of timidity, but a spirit of power, of love and of self-discipline (2 Timothy 1:7).
- **Culturally Relevant**
  ". . . men of Issachar, who understood the times and knew what Israel should do . . ." (1 Chronicles 12:32).*

CMDA Statment of Faith

WE BELIEVE
In the divine inspiration, integrity, and final
authority of the Bible as the Word of God.

In the unique Deity of our Lord Jesus Christ.

In the representative and substitutionary sacrificial death of our
Lord Jesus Christ as the necessary atonement for our sins.

In the presence and power of the Holy Spirit in the work of regeneration.

In the resurrection of the crucified body of our Lord, and the blessed hope,
His personal return.

In the bodily resurrection of the just and unjust, the everlasting
blessedness of the saved and the everlasting punishment of the lost.

Educator of the Year Award

The Educator of the Year Award recognizes outstanding achievement in the area of medical or dental education. In particular, recipients of this award must demonstrate:

- an ability to instill in students a desire for professional excellence, lifelong learning, ethical integrity, and compassion for the suffering;

- unquestioned personal integrity and superior professional competence;

- a commitment to biblical truth and the integration of faith and practice.

RECIPIENTS OF THE EDUCATOR OF THE YEAR AWARD

1996 William P. Wilson, M.D.
1997 Robin J. Catlin, M.D.
1998 Dr. & Mrs. Joe S. McIlhaney, Jr.
1999 Drs. Charles & Lorraine Kelley
2000 Dr. & Mrs. Walter Larimore
2001 Dr. & Mrs. John Crouch

President's Heritage Award

The President's Heritage Award is given to individuals who have contributed greatly to CMDA.

RECIPIENTS OF THE PRESIDENT'S HERITAGE AWARD

1999 Donald F. Westra, J.D.
2000 Gerald Swim
2001 Rev. Marti Ensign

Missionary of the Year Award

The Missionary of the Year Award is presented to a missionary doctor who:

- personifies the qualities of a missionary; namely, love for and passion for reaching unbelievers with the Gospel, an attitude of humility and service, and a courageous and persevering faith;

- demonstrates outstanding effectiveness in ministry, which may or may not be measured in terms of individuals won to the faith;

- inspires others to develop a heart for missions and to serve as full-time or short-term missionaries.

RECIPIENTS OF THE MISSIONARY OF THE YEAR AWARD

1995 Walter B. Hull, M.D.
1996 David S. Topazian, D.D.S.
1997 Harold P. Adolph, M.D.
1998 Carolyn Klaus, M.D.
1999 Dr. & Mrs. Robert Foster
2000 Dr. & Mrs. Daniel Fountain
2001 Dr. & Mrs. Bill Barnett

Servant of Christ Award

In 1972, the Board of Trustees of the Christian Medical Society established the "Man of the Year" award, later changed to the Servant of Christ award. This award was to honor distinguished physicians and dentists whose careers blended well the attributes of committed Christians and competent doctors.

"The designee selected is to exemplify an additional characteristic, namely, a remarkable commitment to excellence in the fields of medical missions, clinical research, patient care, academics or medical ethics," the guidelines read. "This award is given when, in the judgment of the Trustees, the contributions of such a person are called to their attention and merit recognition. Though honors and

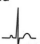

awards in this life may have only temporal significance, nonetheless, they can mark the consensus of responsible peer review that wishes to recognize the remarkable careers some have achieved under the grace of God. To recognize these is to remind students that worthy role models do exist in the Christian medical and dental communities."

The place of service is not the most important factor. But what is important is the servant-leadership lifestyle demonstrating the clear priorities of Christian discipleship, the professional and spiritual integrity of service, the personal quality of truly caring for others, and the sense of ultimate loyalty to Jesus Christ.

A towel and basin—a symbol of Christian humility and service—was chosen as the "trophy."

RECIPIENTS OF THE SERVANT OF CHRIST AWARD
1972 Ernest J. Gregory, M.D.
1973 Paul E. Adolph, M.D.
1974-76 No awards given
1977 Gustav A. Hemwall, M.D.
1978 No award given
1979 Denis Burkitt, M.D.
1980 Ralph Blocksma, M.D.
1981 P. Kenneth Gieser, M.D.
1982 Paul W. Brand, M.D.
1983 Theodora Johnson, M.D.
1984 No award given
1985 Dr. and Mrs. Douglas Harper
1986 John Robert Brobeck, M.D.
1987 Dr. & Mrs. Norval Christy
1988 Drs. David & Martha Stewart
1989 Dr. & Mrs. Ernest Steury
1990 C. Everett Koop, M.D.
1991 William J. Johnson, M.D.
1992 Viggo B. Olsen, M.D.
1993 John D. Frame, M.D.
1994 Dr. & Mrs. Robert Rodriguez
1995 Dr. & Mrs. Peter A. Boelens
1996 Dr. & Mrs. Robert Schindler
1997 Dr. & Mrs. Marvin Jewell
1998 Drs. Tom & Cynthia Hale
1999 Dr. & Mrs. Jack Hough
2000 Dr. & Mrs. Robert Kingsbury
2001 Dr. & Mrs. David Topazian

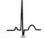

The David L. Stewart, M.D., Lecture Series

Lecturers Honored by the Commission on Medical/Dental Education

1990 Ernest Steury, M.D.
1991 Paul Brand, M.D.
1992 Birch Rambo, M.D.
1993 Norval Christy, M.D.
1994 Helen M. Roseveare, M.B.B.Ch.
1995 John R. Harris, M.B.B.Ch., D.T.M.
1996 Samuel R. J. Cannata, Jr., M.D.
1997 Howard F. Moffett, M.D.
1998 Daniel E. Fountain, M.D.
1999 Carl W. Friedericks. M.D.
2000 Robert S. Schindler, M.D., F.A.C.S.
2001 James D. Miller, D.D.S., M.A., M.A.G.D.

General or Executive Directors

1951-65 J. Raymond Knighton, Jr. – General Director
1965-69 Walter O. Spitzer, M.D. – General Director
1969-71 Christopher Reilly, M.D. – CMS President & Interim General Director
1971-79 Haddon Robinson, D.Th., Ph.D. – General Director
1979-81 Joseph Bayly – General Director
1980-82 Donald F. Westra, J.D. – Executive Director
1981-82 Arthur H. Svedberg, M.D. – Acting General Director
1982-83 L. Arden Almquist, M.D. – General Director
1983-84 Donald F. Westra, J.D. – General Director
1984-87 Edwin Blum, D.Th., Ph.D. – General Director
1987 Mayo D. Gilson, M.D. – CMS President & Interim General Director
1987-93 Hal Habecker, D. Min. – General Director
1993-94 Robert Schiedt, M.D. – CMDS President & Interim General Director
1994-Present David Stevens, M.D. – Executive Director

Past Presidents of CMDA

1946 C. James Krafft, M.D.
1947 Vernoy A. Reihmer, M.D.
1948 John Elsen, M.D.
1949 Richard E. Scheel, M.D.
1950 Dean B. Smith, M.D.
1951 Howard Hamlin, M.D.
1952 William H. Whiteley, M.D.
1953-54 P. Kenneth Gieser, M.D.
1954-55 J. Winslow Smith, M.D.
1955-56 John S. Hyde, M.D.
1956-57 Gustav A. Hemwall, M.D.
1957-58 Delburt H. Nelson, M.D.
1958-59 Ralph Blocksma, M.D.
1959-60 P. Kenneth Gieser, M.D.
1960-61 William A. Johnson, M.D.
1961-62 William H. Whitely, M.D.
1962-63 Reynold J. Gottlieb, M.D.
1963-64 C. James Krafft, M.D.
1964-65 Martin H. Andrews, M.D.
1965-66 P. Kenneth Gieser, M.D.
1966 C. Markham Berry, M.D.
1966-67 Paul J. Jorden, M.D.
1967-69 Arthur H. Svedberg, M.D.
1969-71 Christopher T. Reilly, M.D.
1971-73 Gustav A. Hemwall, M.D.
1973-75 John H. Dawson, M.D.
1975-77 Marvin R. Jewell, Jr., M.D.
1977-79 John H. Lindberg, M.D.
1979-81 Leonard W. Ritzmann, M.D.
1981-83 James A. Petersen, M.D.
1983-85 Curtis C. Drevets, M.D.
1985-87 Robert S. Schindler, M.D.
1987-89 Mayo D. Gilson, M.D.
1989-91 David S. Topazian, D.D.S.
1991-93 Robert J. Kingsbury, M.D.
1993-95 Robert B. Scheidt, M.D.
1995-97 Donald K. Wood, M.D.
1997-99 Dorothy Barbo, M.D.
1999-2001 Robert F. Agnew, M.D.

Current:
2001-2003   Alva B. Weir III, M.D.

CMDA Field Staff [2002]

Regional Directors
Scott Boyles, M.Div., Northeast Regional Director
Allan Harmer, Th.M., Midwest Regional Director
Doug Hornok, Th.M., Central Regional Director
Michael McLaughlin, M.Div., Western Regional Director

Area Directors
Stan Cobb, D.D.S., Dallas Area Director
Brooks Goodgame, M.Div., Chicago Area Director
Lem Howard, M.Div., Virginia Area Director
Roger Matkin, D.Min., San Antonio Area Director
Ken Nippert, M.Div., Memphis Area Director
Bill Pearson, B.S., Harvard Medical School Area Director
Scott Phillips, M.Div., Northeast Ohio Area Director
Andy Sanders, M.D., Augusta (Georgia) Area Director
Jimmy Turner, B.A., Jackson (Mississippi) Area Director

CMDA Ministries at a Glance

Evangelism
Saline Solution Training (conferences and video)
Pre-evangelism events
Exhibits at major medical meetings

Discipleship
Local Chapters
Student Chapters on 160 campuses
Local Councils directing local outreaches
Local and regional retreats
Regional and national conferences
Commissions
Women in Medicine
Singles
Marriage
Malpractice

Leadership Training – student and graduate leaders

Mentor Match – matching first year residents with graduate doctors

Service
Global Health Outreach
Commission on International Medical Education Affairs
Domestic Mission Commission

Resident and Student Mission Scholarship Funds
Steury Medical School Scholarship Fund
International Christian Medical & Dental Association affiliation
Discounted phone service supporting GHO outreach
CMDA credit card supporting commission ministries
CMDA Speakers Bureau

Equipping
Today's Christian Doctor Magazine
Christian Doctor's Digest Audio Tapes

Commissions
    Continuing Medical & Dental Education for missionary doctors
    Medical Malpractice Commission
    Ethics Commission

Paul Tournier Institute – producing curriculum and other resources
Co-publishing books with Zondervan Corporation for the church/public
The Scan – monthly publication of key articles for medical missionaries
Web site: http://www.cmdahome.org
CMDA Placement Service
Life & Health Resources
Sight and Sound Resources – videos, tapes, CD's and other resources
Stewardship Services – estate planning assistance, donor advised funds

Voice
Public Service Announcements
News Releases to secular and Christian media
Media interviews
Bioethics Resource Kits
Ethics Hotline
Media Training
News & Views e-mail updates
Congressional Testimony
Professional advice to Congress and other organizations
News Conferences
Washington Bureau

Note: All biblical references in this appendix are from the New International Version (NIV).